ANATOMY & PATHOLOGY 5th Edition

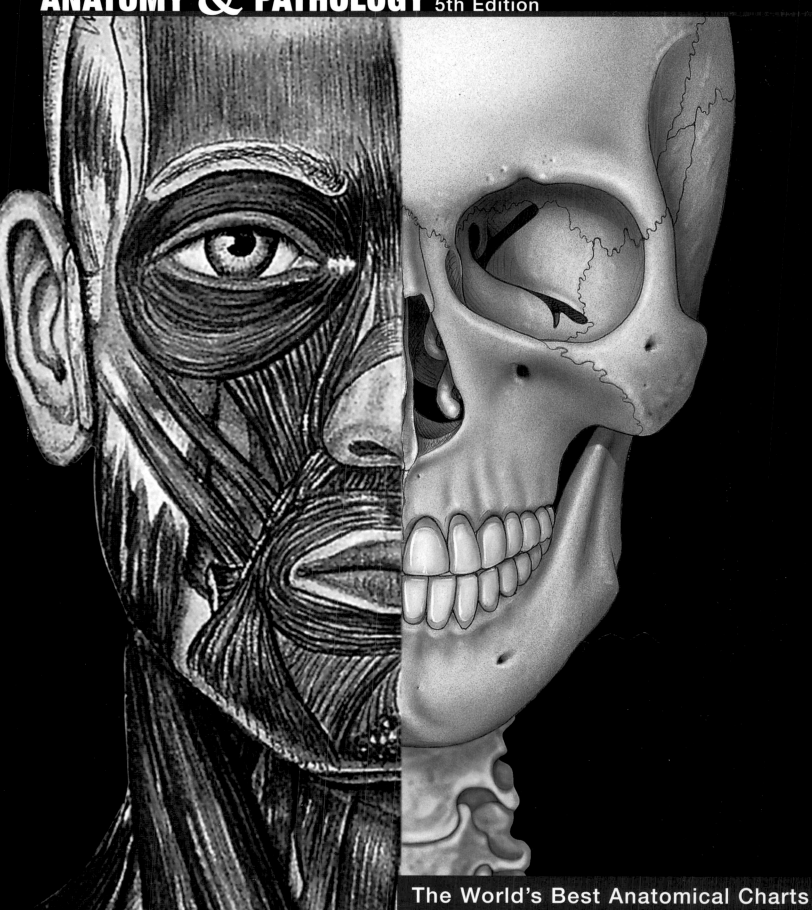

The World's Best Anatomical Charts

CONTENTS

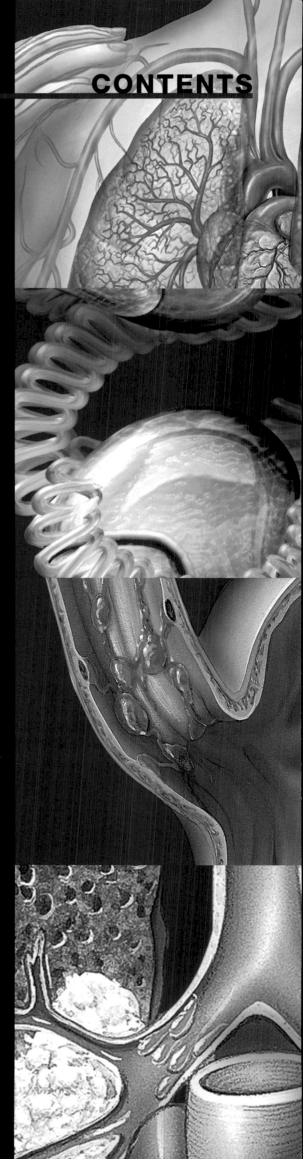

Copyright ©1993, 1995, 2000, 2005, 2008 Wolters Kluwer | Lippincott Williams & Wilkins
Health

Published by **Anatomical Chart Company, Skokie, IL USA**
5th Edition
ISBN 10: 0-7817-7356-3
ISBN 13: 978-0-7817-7356-0   Library of Congress Control Number: 2007922821

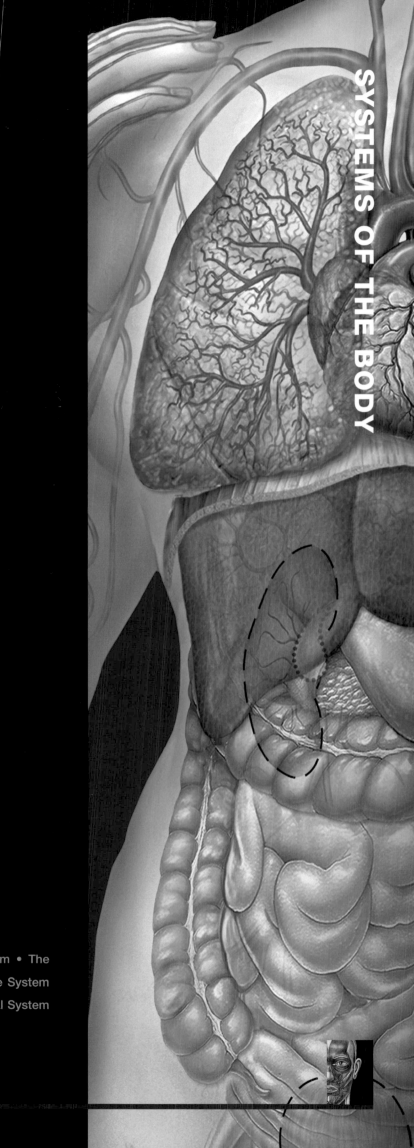

SYSTEMS OF THE BODY

The Digestive System

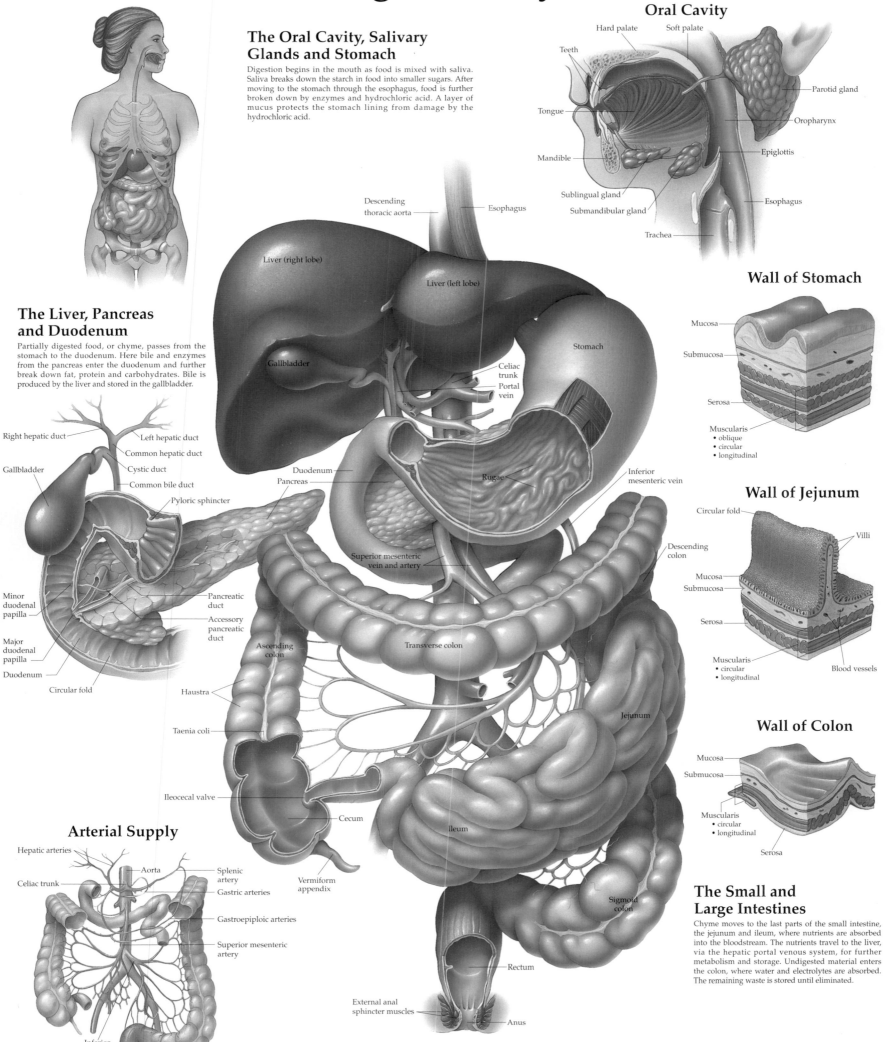

The Oral Cavity, Salivary Glands and Stomach

Digestion begins in the mouth as food is mixed with saliva. Saliva breaks down the starch in food into smaller sugars. After moving to the stomach through the esophagus, food is further broken down by enzymes and hydrochloric acid. A layer of mucus protects the stomach lining from damage by the hydrochloric acid.

Oral Cavity

Hard palate · Soft palate · Teeth · Tongue · Mandible · Parotid gland · Oropharynx · Epiglottis · Sublingual gland · Submandibular gland · Esophagus · Trachea

The Liver, Pancreas and Duodenum

Partially digested food, or chyme, passes from the stomach to the duodenum. Here bile and enzymes from the pancreas enter the duodenum and further break down fat, protein and carbohydrates. Bile is produced by the liver and stored in the gallbladder.

Right hepatic duct · Left hepatic duct · Common hepatic duct · Cystic duct · Gallbladder · Common bile duct · Pyloric sphincter · Minor duodenal papilla · Major duodenal papilla · Duodenum · Circular fold · Pancreatic duct · Accessory pancreatic duct

Descending thoracic aorta · Esophagus · Liver (right lobe) · Liver (left lobe) · Gallbladder · Stomach · Celiac trunk · Portal vein · Duodenum · Pancreas · Rugae · Inferior mesenteric vein · Superior mesenteric vein and artery

Wall of Stomach

Mucosa · Submucosa · Serosa · Muscularis · oblique · circular · longitudinal

Wall of Jejunum

Circular fold · Villi · Mucosa · Submucosa · Serosa · Muscularis · circular · longitudinal · Blood vessels

Wall of Colon

Mucosa · Submucosa · Muscularis · circular · longitudinal · Serosa

Descending colon · Transverse colon · Ascending colon · Haustra · Taenia coli · Ileocecal valve · Cecum · Jejunum · Ileum · Vermiform appendix · Sigmoid colon · Rectum · External anal sphincter muscles · Anus

Arterial Supply

Hepatic arteries · Celiac trunk · Aorta · Splenic artery · Gastric arteries · Gastroepiploic arteries · Superior mesenteric artery · Inferior mesenteric artery

The Small and Large Intestines

Chyme moves to the last parts of the small intestine, the jejunum and ileum, where nutrients are absorbed into the bloodstream. The nutrients travel to the liver, via the hepatic portal venous system, for further metabolism and storage. Undigested material enters the colon, where water and electrolytes are absorbed. The remaining waste is stored until eliminated.

©2008 Wolters Kluwer | Lippincott Williams & Wilkins | Published by Anatomical Chart Company, Skokie, IL

The Endocrine System

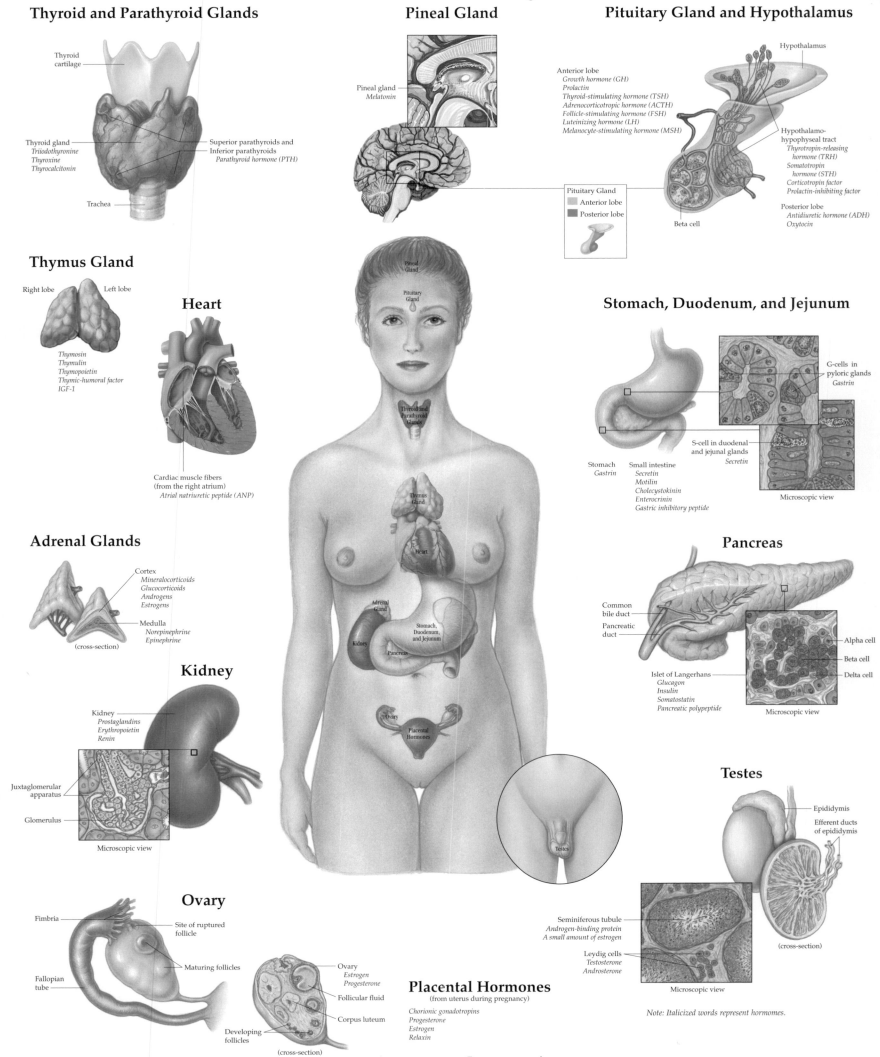

Thyroid and Parathyroid Glands

Thyroid cartilage

Thyroid gland
Triiodothyronine
Thyroxine
Thyrocalcitonin

Superior parathyroids and
Inferior parathyroids
Parathyroid hormone (PTH)

Trachea

Pineal Gland

Pineal gland
Melatonin

Pituitary Gland and Hypothalamus

Hypothalamus

Anterior lobe
Growth hormone (GH)
Prolactin
Thyroid-stimulating hormone (TSH)
Adrenocorticotropic hormone (ACTH)
Follicle-stimulating hormone (FSH)
Luteinizing hormone (LH)
Melanocyte-stimulating hormone (MSH)

Hypothalamo-
hypophyseal tract
Thyrotropin-releasing
hormone (TRH)
Somatotropin
hormone (STH)
Corticotropin factor
Prolactin-inhibiting factor

Posterior lobe
Antidiuretic hormone (ADH)
Oxytocin

Beta cell

Pituitary Gland
Anterior lobe
Posterior lobe

Thymus Gland

Right lobe   Left lobe

Thymosin
Thymulin
Thymopoietin
Thymic-humoral factor
IGF-1

Heart

Cardiac muscle fibers
(from the right atrium)
Atrial natriuretic peptide (ANP)

Adrenal Glands

Cortex
Mineralocorticoids
Glucocorticoids
Androgens
Estrogens

Medulla
Norepinephrine
Epinephrine

(cross-section)

Kidney

Kidney
Prostaglandins
Erythropoietin
Renin

Juxtaglomerular
apparatus

Glomerulus

Microscopic view

Stomach, Duodenum, and Jejunum

G-cells in
pyloric glands
Gastrin

S-cell in duodenal
and jejunal glands
Secretin

Stomach
Gastrin

Small intestine
Secretin
Motilin
Cholecystokinin
Enterocrinin
Gastric inhibitory peptide

Microscopic view

Pancreas

Common
bile duct

Pancreatic
duct

Alpha cell
Beta cell
Delta cell

Islet of Langerhans
Glucagon
Insulin
Somatostatin
Pancreatic polypeptide

Microscopic view

Testes

Epididymis

Efferent ducts
of epididymis

Seminiferous tubule
Androgen-binding protein
A small amount of estrogen

Leydig cells
Testosterone
Androsterone

(cross-section)

Microscopic view

Ovary

Fimbria

Site of ruptured
follicle

Maturing follicles

Fallopian
tube

Ovary
Estrogen
Progesterone

Follicular fluid

Corpus luteum

Developing
follicles

(cross-section)

Placental Hormones
(from uterus during pregnancy)

Chorionic gonadotropins
Progesterone
Estrogen
Relaxin

Note: Italicized words represent hormones.

Labels on body figure: Pineal Gland, Pituitary Gland, Thyroid and Parathyroid Glands, Thymus Gland, Heart, Adrenal Gland, Stomach, Duodenum, and Jejunum, Pancreas, Kidney, Ovary, Placental Hormones, Testes

©2008 Wolters Kluwer Health | Lippincott Williams & Wilkins I Published by Anatomical Chart Company, Skokie, IL

Ovum
(Unfertilized)
100-150μm diameter

Nucleus
Nucleolus
Ooplasm
Zona pellucida
Polar body
Corona radiata

Ovary, Fallopian Tube, Uterus and Vagina

Suspensory ligament of ovary
Fallopian tube
Isthmus
Fundus of uterus
Ampulla
Infundibulum
Fimbria
Abdominal opening of fallopian tube
Secondary oocyte
Corpus luteum
Ovarian ligament
Ovary
Vesicular appendix
Cavity of uterus
Broad ligament
Uterus:
Perimetrium
Myometrium
Endometrium
Internal uterine opening
Cervix
Cervical canal
External uterine opening
Vagina
Labium minus

The Female Pelvic Organs
(Sagittal section)

L5
Suspensory ligament of ovary
Ovary
Fallopian tube
Ovarian ligament
Round ligament
Median umbilical ligament
Urinary bladder
Pubic symphysis
Urethra
Clitoris
Prepuce of clitoris
Urethral orifice
Labium minus
Labium majus
Vaginal orifice
Sacrum
Ureter
Rectum
Uterus
Posterior fornix of vagina
Rectouterine pouch
Cervix
Levator ani muscle
Vagina
Anus

The Female Perineum

Pubic symphysis
Prepuce
Clitoris:
Body
Glans
Crus
Urethral orifice
Ischiocavernous muscle
Labium majus
Labium minus
Bulbospongiosus muscle
Vaginal orifice
Deep transverse perineal muscle
Ischial tuberosity
Pudendal nerve
Levator ani muscle
Anus
External anal sphincter
Gluteus maximus muscle

Ovary

Mature graafian follicle
Antrum filled with liquor folliculi
Expulsion of secondary oocyte
Primary oocyte
Developing follicles
Corpus luteum

Uterus

Ovulation
Uterine gland
Venous lacunae
Endometrium:
Stratum functionale
Endometrial vein
Spiral artery
Stratum basale
Myometrium
Basal artery
Arcuate artery

Day 0   4   14   26   28
Menstrual phase
Proliferative phase
Secretory phase
Premenstrual phase

The Menstrual Cycle
The menstrual cycle occurs during the reproductive period from puberty through menopause in response to rhythmic variations of hormones. The endometrial lining of the uterus proliferates in preparation for implantation of a fertilized egg. In the absence of pregnancy the lining is shed with some bleeding through the vagina.

Menopause
Menopause, the gradual interruption and cessation of menstrual cycles, occurs at about 45 to 50 years of age. It is associated with the depletion of oocytes in the ovary and subsequent decline of estrogen levels.

©2008 Wolters Kluwer Health | Lippincott Williams & Wilkins | Published by Anatomical Chart Company, Skokie, IL

ALLERGIC RESPONSE

THE IMMUNE SYSTEM

Allergens:
Most allergens are relatively small, highly soluble proteins that are carried on dry particles such as pollen and mite feces.

The Initial Encounter:

1st TH2 cells are activated and release cytokines that stimulate B-lymphocytes.

Antigen Presenting Cell (APC):
A macrophage-like cell that is capable of taking up allergens, processing, and packaging them so that the small pieces are placed together with MHC class-II molecules in order to express them on their surface and present them to T cells.

Allergic Reactions- Immediate and Late Reaction

Immediate reaction is a result of chemical mediators, including histamine, prostaglandins, and other preformed and newly synthesized mediators, that cause a rapid increase in vasopermeability, vasodilation, gastric acid secretion, itching, and smooth muscle contraction.

Late reaction can occur within hours of an acute allergic reaction. Activated mast cells and basophils release mediators, including prostaglandins, leukotrienes, chemokines, and cytokines, which cause inflammation; these mediators in turn call upon other leukocytes, including eosinophils and TH2 lymphocytes, to the site of inflammation. Late-phase reactions are associated with a second phase of smooth muscle contraction mediated by T-cells and tissue remodeling such as smooth muscle hypertrophy and hyperplasia.

T-lymphocytes:
There are two main types of T-cells called T-helper cells or Th cells that respond to antigens:

Th1 lymphocytes – release cytokines that drive up inflammation in order to destroy invading pathogens (infection fighters).

Th2 lymphocytes – release a different set of cytokines that drive B cells and antibody formation (allergy promoters).

Cytokines:
A set of proteins produced by lymphocytes and macrophages in response to an inflammation such as an allergen.

IgE:
IgE is an antibody produced by plasma cells (mature B-lymphocytes) located in lymph nodes and at the sites of allergic reactions. It binds to mast cells and basophils, and activates eosinophils; IgE helps these cells to "home" in on the offending antigens. People who are more prone to allergic reactions typically have higher levels of IgE in their bodies.

B-lymphocytes:
The precursors of tiny "antibody factories" (plasma cells) that produce antibodies to help remove foreign substances upon stimulation by Th2 cells.

Basophils:
Basophils are also called to the sites of allergic reactions causing inflammation and tissue damage.

Upon activation, basophils release:

- **HISTAMINE** – a substance derived from the amino acid histidine. It causes an immediate increase in local blood flow and vessel permeability.

- **IL-4** – a cytokine that helps in the development of allergies.

Primed:

2nd Once "sensitized" or "primed", B-lymphocytes differentiate into plasma cells. These cells produce IgE antibodies that bind to granulocytes (basophils, eosinophils) and mast cells, preparing them to bind to the allergen upon a second exposure.

Eosinophils:
Eosinophils are granulocytic leukocytes that originate in bone marrow. They cause inflammation and tissue damage in allergic reactions.

Activation and degranulation of eosinophils is strictly regulated to prevent inappropriate toxic responses. Eosinophils, basophils, and mast cells can interact with each other.

Activation and Regulation of Eosinophils:

1. Eosinophils have a high threshold for the release of their granule contents when inactive.

2. Cytokines such as IL-5 are released when specialized T cells (TH2) are activated; these cytokines increase the production of eosinophils in the bone marrow and their release into the circulation. After activation of eosinophils by cytokines and chemokines, this threshold decreases.

3. Eosinophil degranulation releases major basic protein, which causes degranulation of mast cells and basophils; this causes an increase of IgE receptors on the surface leading to tissue damage.

Activated:

3rd When the specific allergen comes into contact again, the IgE, now transfixed on the surface of reactive cells, leads to an explosion releasing a number of chemicals (preformed mediators) that produce the allergic reaction which we can see and feel.

Mast Cells:
Mast cells are highly specialized. They are very similar to the basophils except that mast cells do not circulate in the blood; they are present in the tissues.

Mast cells release a variety of preformed inflammatory mediators:

- **HISTAMINE** causes an immediate increase in local blood flow and vessel permeability.

- **ENZYMES** cause tissue destruction.

- **TUMOR NECROSIS FACTOR (TNF)** promote the flow of inflammatory leukocytes and lymphocytes into tissues.

Upon activation, mast cells synthesize and release chemokines and lipid mediators (prostaglandins, leukotrienes).

- **LIPID MEDIATORS** cause smooth muscle contraction, increase vascular permeability, and increase mucus secretion. They also induce the influx and activation of leukocytes, which contribute to the late phase of the allergic response.

- **PROSTAGLANDIN D2** activates or signals eosinophils, basophils and TH2 lymphocytes.

The Lymphatic System

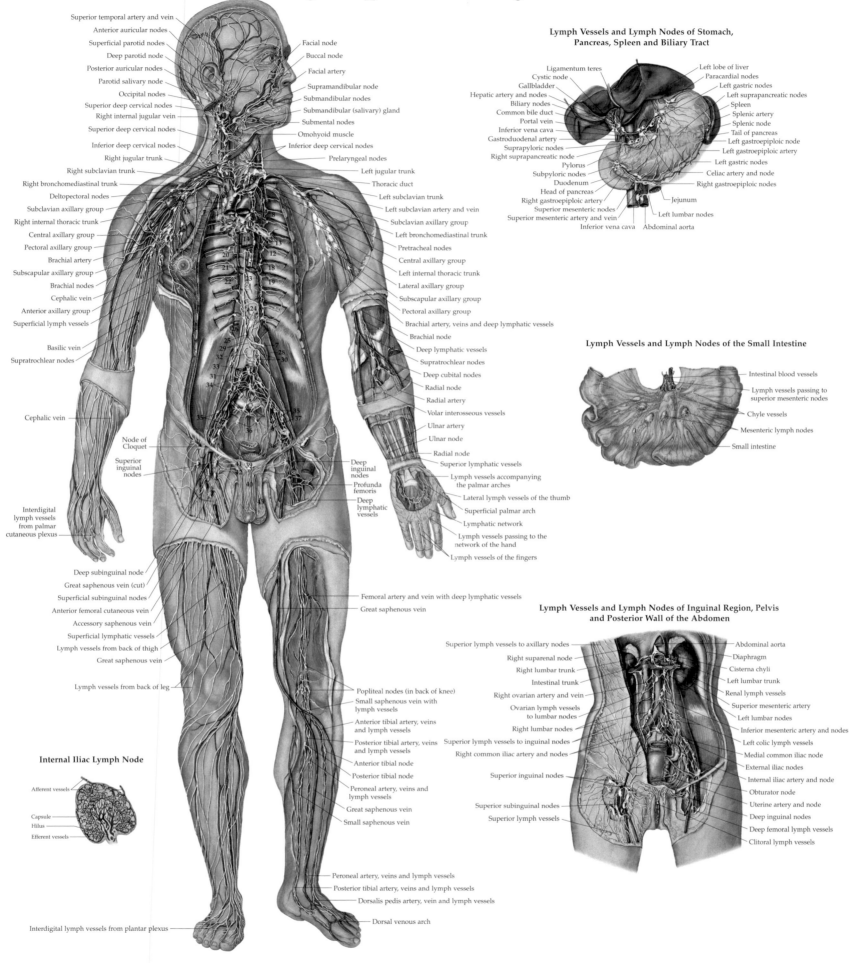

Superior temporal artery and vein
Anterior auricular nodes
Superficial parotid nodes
Deep parotid node
Posterior auricular nodes
Parotid salivary node
Occipital nodes
Superior deep cervical nodes
Right internal jugular vein
Superior deep cervical nodes
Inferior deep cervical nodes
Right jugular trunk
Right subclavian trunk
Right bronchomediastinal trunk
Deltopectoral nodes
Subclavian axillary group
Right internal thoracic trunk
Central axillary group
Pectoral axillary group
Brachial artery
Subscapular axillary group
Brachial nodes
Cephalic vein
Anterior axillary group
Superficial lymph vessels
Basilic vein
Supratrochlear nodes
Cephalic vein
Node of Cloquet
Superior inguinal nodes
Interdigital lymph vessels from palmar cutaneous plexus

Facial node
Buccal node
Facial artery
Supramandibular node
Submandibular nodes
Submandibular (salivary) gland
Submental nodes
Omohyoid muscle
Inferior deep cervical nodes
Prelaryngeal nodes
Left jugular trunk
Thoracic duct
Left subclavian trunk
Left subclavian artery and vein
Subclavian axillary group
Left bronchomediastinal trunk
Pretracheal nodes
Central axillary group
Left internal thoracic trunk
Lateral axillary group
Subscapular axillary group
Pectoral axillary group
Brachial artery, veins and deep lymphatic vessels
Brachial node
Deep lymphatic vessels
Supratrochlear nodes
Deep cubital nodes
Radial node
Radial artery
Volar interosseous vessels
Ulnar artery
Ulnar vein
Radial node
Superior lymphatic vessels
Deep inguinal nodes
Profunda femoris
Deep lymphatic vessels
Lymph vessels accompanying the palmar arches
Lateral lymph vessels of the thumb
Superficial palmar arch
Lymphatic network
Lymph vessels passing to the network of the hand
Lymph vessels of the fingers

Deep subinguinal node
Great saphenous vein (cut)
Superficial subinguinal nodes
Anterior femoral cutaneous vein
Accessory saphenous vein
Superficial lymphatic vessels
Lymph vessels from back of thigh
Great saphenous vein
Lymph vessels from back of leg

Femoral artery and vein with deep lymphatic vessels
Great saphenous vein

Popliteal nodes (in back of knee)
Small saphenous vein with lymph vessels
Anterior tibial artery, veins and lymph vessels
Posterior tibial artery, veins and lymph vessels
Anterior tibial node
Posterior tibial node
Peroneal artery, veins and lymph vessels
Great saphenous vein
Small saphenous vein

Peroneal artery, veins and lymph vessels
Posterior tibial artery, veins and lymph vessels
Dorsalis pedis artery, vein and lymph vessels
Dorsal venous arch

Interdigital lymph vessels from plantar plexus

Lymph Vessels and Lymph Nodes of Stomach, Pancreas, Spleen and Biliary Tract

Ligamentum teres
Cystic node
Gallbladder
Hepatic artery and nodes
Biliary nodes
Common bile duct
Portal vein
Inferior vena cava
Gastroduodenal artery
Suprapyloric nodes
Right suprapancreatic node
Pylorus
Subpyloric nodes
Duodenum
Head of pancreas
Right gastroepiploic artery
Superior mesenteric nodes
Superior mesenteric artery and vein
Inferior vena cava

Left lobe of liver
Paracardial nodes
Left gastric nodes
Left suprapancreatic nodes
Spleen
Splenic artery
Splenic node
Tail of pancreas
Left gastroepiploic node
Left gastroepiploic artery
Left gastric nodes
Celiac artery and node
Right gastroepiploic nodes
Jejunum
Left lumbar nodes
Abdominal aorta

Lymph Vessels and Lymph Nodes of the Small Intestine

Intestinal blood vessels
Lymph vessels passing to superior mesenteric nodes
Chyle vessels
Mesenteric lymph nodes
Small intestine

Lymph Vessels and Lymph Nodes of Inguinal Region, Pelvis and Posterior Wall of the Abdomen

Superior lymph vessels to axillary nodes
Right suprarenal node
Right lumbar trunk
Intestinal trunk
Right ovarian artery and vein
Ovarian lymph vessels to lumbar nodes
Right lumbar nodes
Superior lymph vessels to inguinal nodes
Right common iliac artery and nodes
Superior inguinal nodes
Superior subinguinal nodes
Superior lymph vessels

Abdominal aorta
Diaphragm
Cisterna chyli
Left lumbar trunk
Renal lymph vessels
Superior mesenteric artery
Inferior mesenteric artery and nodes
Left colic lymph vessels
Medial common iliac node
External iliac nodes
Internal iliac artery and node
Obturator node
Uterine artery and node
Deep inguinal nodes
Deep femoral lymph vessels
Clitoral lymph vessels

Internal Iliac Lymph Node

Afferent vessels
Capsule
Hilus
Efferent vessels

1. Right brachiocephalic vein
2. Left brachiocephalic vein
3. Left common carotid artery
4. Anterior superior mediastinal nodes
5. Superior vena cava
6. Right cardiac lymph branch
7. Internal thoracic node
8. Node of ligamentum arteriosum
9. Right bronchus
10. Left bronchus
11. Right tracheobronchial nodes
12. Left tracheobronchial nodes
13. Right and left bronchopulmonary nodes
14. Esophagus
15. Internal thoracic lymph vessel ending in subclavicular nodes
16. Interpectoral nodes
17. Lymph vessels from deep part of breast
18. Posterior mediastinal nodes
19. Intercostal nodes and lymph vessels
20. Azygos vein
21. Thoracic duct
22. Thoracic aorta
23. Hemiazygos vein
24. Descending right and left intercostal lymph trunks
25. Cisterna chyli
26. Right crus of diaphragm
27. Intestinal trunk
28. Psoas major muscle
29. Right and left lumbar trunks
30. Lumbar nodes
31. Testicular lymph vessels
32. Retroaortic node (lumbar nodes)
33. Preaortic node (lumbar nodes)
34. Common iliac nodes
35. Internal iliac artery and nodes
36. Sacral nodes
37. Lymph vessels to internal iliac nodes
38. Obturator vessels and nerve
39. Presymphysial node
40. Collecting lymph vessels from glans penis
41. Superior lymph vessels from the penis
42. Lymph vessels from the scrotum
43. Lymph vessels of testis and epididymus

©2008 Wolters Kluwer Health | Lippincott Williams & Wilkins | Published by Anatomical Chart Company, Skokie, IL

The Male Reproductive System

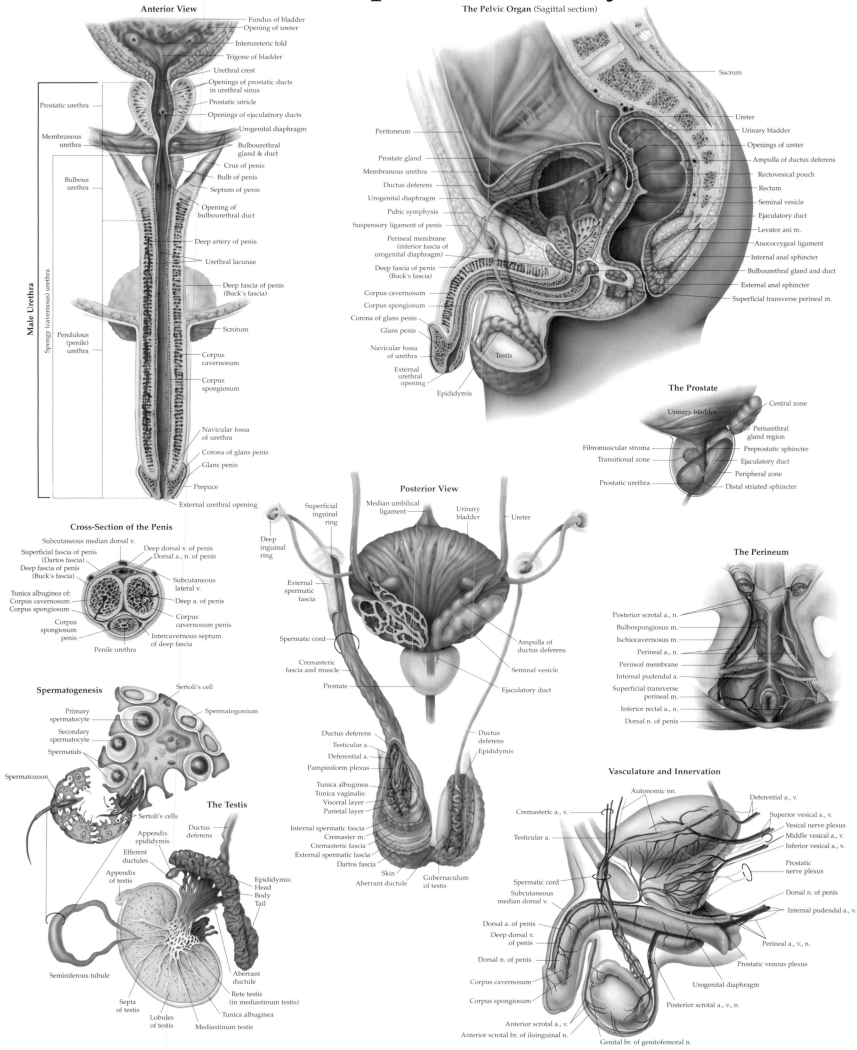

Anterior View

- Fundus of bladder
- Opening of ureter
- Interureteric fold
- Trigone of bladder
- Urethral crest
- Openings of prostatic ducts in urethral sinus
- Prostatic utricle
- Openings of ejaculatory ducts
- Urogenital diaphragm
- Bulbourethral gland & duct
- Crus of penis
- Bulb of penis
- Septum of penis
- Opening of bulbourethral duct
- Deep artery of penis
- Urethral lacunae
- Deep fascia of penis (Buck's fascia)
- Scrotum
- Corpus cavernosum
- Corpus spongiosum
- Navicular fossa of urethra
- Corona of glans penis
- Glans penis
- Prepuce
- External urethral opening

Prostatic urethra
Membranous urethra
Bulbous urethra
Pendulous (penile) urethra
Male Urethra
Spongy (cavernous) urethra

The Pelvic Organ (Sagittal section)

- Sacrum
- Ureter
- Urinary bladder
- Openings of ureter
- Ampulla of ductus deferens
- Rectovesical pouch
- Rectum
- Seminal vesicle
- Ejaculatory duct
- Levator ani m.
- Anococcygeal ligament
- Internal anal sphincter
- Bulbourethral gland and duct
- External anal sphincter
- Superficial transverse perineal m.
- Peritoneum
- Prostate gland
- Membranous urethra
- Ductus deferens
- Urogenital diaphragm
- Pubic symphysis
- Suspensory ligament of penis
- Perineal membrane (inferior fascia of urogenital diaphragm)
- Deep fascia of penis (Buck's fascia)
- Corpus cavernosum
- Corpus spongiosum
- Corona of glans penis
- Glans penis
- Navicular fossa of urethra
- External urethral opening
- Testis
- Epididymis

The Prostate

- Central zone
- Periurethral gland region
- Preprostatic sphincter
- Ejaculatory duct
- Peripheral zone
- Distal striated sphincter
- Urinary bladder
- Fibromuscular stroma
- Transitional zone
- Prostatic urethra

Cross-Section of the Penis

- Subcutaneous median dorsal v.
- Superficial fascia of penis (Dartos fascia)
- Deep fascia of penis (Buck's fascia)
- Tunica albuginea of: Corpus cavernosum / Corpus spongiosum
- Corpus spongiosum penis
- Penile urethra
- Deep dorsal v. of penis
- Dorsal a., n. of penis
- Subcutaneous lateral v.
- Deep a. of penis
- Corpus cavernosum penis
- Intercavernous septum of deep fascia

Posterior View

- Median umbilical ligament
- Urinary bladder
- Ureter
- Superficial inguinal ring
- Deep inguinal ring
- External spermatic fascia
- Spermatic cord
- Cremasteric fascia and muscle
- Ampulla of ductus deferens
- Seminal vesicle
- Prostate
- Ejaculatory duct

The Perineum

- Posterior scrotal a., n.
- Bulbospongiosus m.
- Ischiocavernosus m.
- Perineal a., n.
- Perineal membrane
- Internal pudendal a.
- Superficial transverse perineal m.
- Inferior rectal a., n.
- Dorsal n. of penis

Spermatogenesis

- Sertoli's cell
- Spermatogonium
- Primary spermatocyte
- Secondary spermatocyte
- Spermatids
- Spermatozoon
- Sertoli's cells

The Testis

- Ductus deferens
- Testicular a.
- Deferential a.
- Pampiniform plexus
- Tunica albuginea
- Tunica vaginalis: Visceral layer / Parietal layer
- Internal spermatic fascia
- Cremaster m.
- Cremasteric fascia
- External spermatic fascia
- Dartos fascia
- Skin
- Aberrant ductule
- Ductus deferens
- Epididymis
- Gubernaculum of testis
- Appendix epididymis
- Efferent ductules
- Appendix of testis
- Epididymis: Head / Body / Tail
- Seminiferous tubule
- Aberrant ductule
- Rete testis (in mediastinum testis)
- Septa of testis
- Tunica albuginea
- Lobules of testis
- Mediastinum testis

Vasculature and Innervation

- Autonomic nn.
- Deferential a., v.
- Superior vesical a., v.
- Vesical nerve plexus
- Middle vesical a., v.
- Inferior vesical a., v.
- Cremasteric a., v.
- Testicular a.
- Prostatic nerve plexus
- Spermatic cord
- Subcutaneous median dorsal v.
- Dorsal n. of penis
- Internal pudendal a., v.
- Dorsal a. of penis
- Deep dorsal v. of penis
- Dorsal n. of penis
- Perineal a., v., n.
- Prostatic venous plexus
- Corpus cavernosum
- Corpus spongiosum
- Urogenital diaphragm
- Posterior scrotal a., v., n.
- Anterior scrotal a., v.
- Anterior scrotal br. of ilioinguinal n.
- Genital br. of genitofemoral n.

©2008 Wolters Kluwer | Lippincott Williams & Wilkins | Published by Anatomical Chart Company, Skokie, IL

The Muscular System

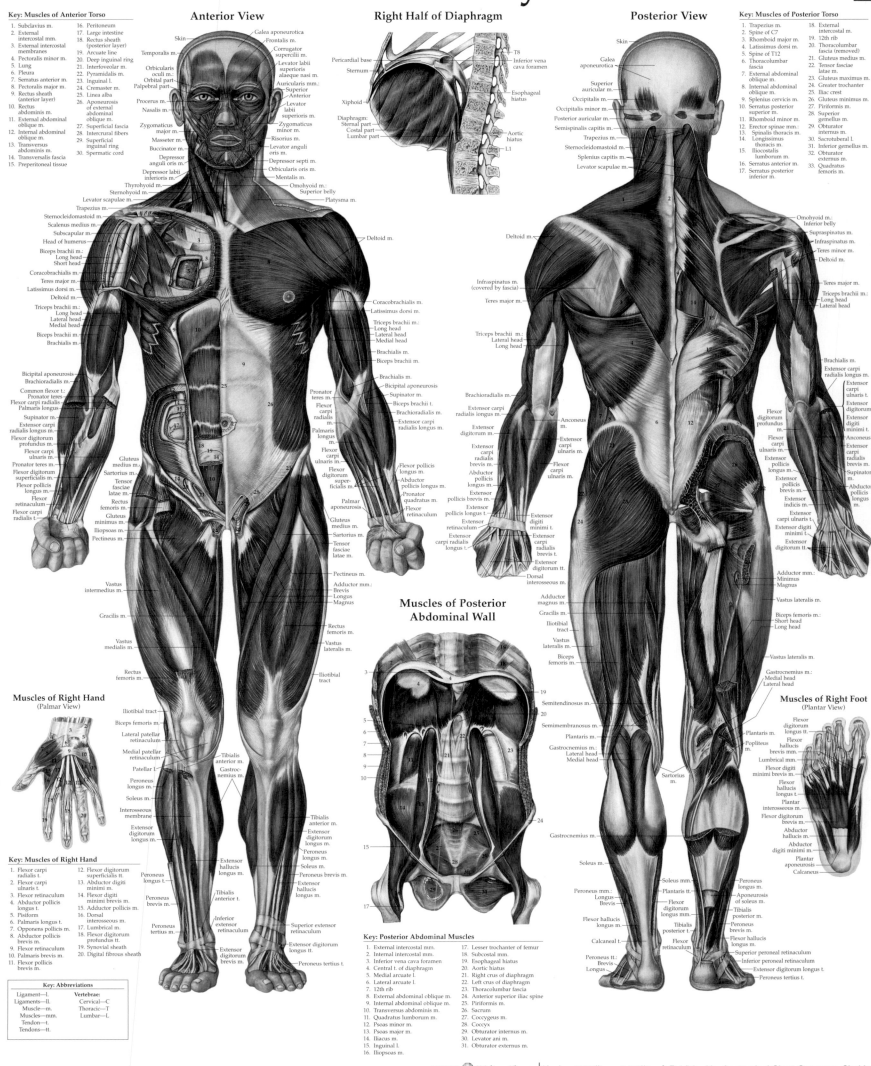

Anterior View

Right Half of Diaphragm

Posterior View

Muscles of Right Hand (Palmar View)

Muscles of Posterior Abdominal Wall

Muscles of Right Foot (Plantar View)

Key: Muscles of Anterior Torso

1. Subclavius m.
2. External intercostal mm.
3. External intercostal membranes
4. Pectoralis minor m.
5. Lung
6. Pleura
7. Serratus anterior m.
8. Pectoralis major m.
9. Rectus sheath (anterior layer)
10. Rectus abdominis m.
11. External abdominal oblique m.
12. Internal abdominal oblique m.
13. Transversus abdominis m.
14. Transversalis fascia
15. Preperitoneal tissue
16. Peritoneum
17. Large intestine
18. Rectus sheath (posterior layer)
19. Arcuate line
20. Deep inguinal ring
21. Interfoveolar m.
22. Inguinal l.
23. Cremaster m.
24. Linea alba
25. Pyramidalis m.
26. Aponeurosis of external abdominal oblique m.
27. Superficial fascia
28. Intercrural fibers
29. Superficial inguinal ring
30. Spermatic cord

Key: Muscles of Posterior Torso

1. Trapezius m.
2. Spine of C7
3. Rhomboid major m.
4. Latissimus dorsi m.
5. Spine of T12
6. Thoracolumbar fascia
7. External abdominal oblique m.
8. Internal abdominal oblique m.
9. Splenius cervicis m.
10. Serratus posterior superior m.
11. Rhomboid minor m.
12. Erector spinae mm.
13. Spinalis thoracis m.
14. Longissimus thoracis m.
15. Iliocostalis lumborum m.
16. Serratus anterior m.
17. Serratus posterior inferior m.
18. External intercostal m.
19. 12th rib
20. Thoracolumbar fascia (removed)
21. Gluteus medius m.
22. Tensor fasciae latae m.
23. Gluteus maximus m.
24. Greater trochanter
25. Iliac crest
26. Gluteus minimus m.
27. Piriformis m.
28. Superior gemellus m.
29. Obturator internus m.
30. Sacrotuberal l.
31. Inferior gemellus m.
32. Obturator externus m.
33. Quadratus femoris m.

Key: Muscles of Right Hand

1. Flexor carpi radialis t.
2. Flexor carpi ulnaris t.
3. Flexor retinaculum
4. Abductor pollicis longus t.
5. Pisiform
6. Palmaris longus t.
7. Opponens pollicis m.
8. Abductor pollicis brevis m.
9. Flexor retinaculum
10. Palmaris brevis m.
11. Flexor pollicis brevis m.
12. Flexor digitorum superficialis tt.
13. Abductor digiti minimi m.
14. Flexor digiti minimi brevis m.
15. Adductor pollicis m.
16. Dorsal interosseous m.
17. Lumbrical m.
18. Flexor digitorum profundus tt.
19. Synovial sheath
20. Digital fibrous sheath

Key: Posterior Abdominal Muscles

1. External intercostal mm.
2. Internal intercostal mm.
3. Inferior vena cava foramen
4. Central t. of diaphragm
5. Medial arcuate l.
6. Lateral arcuate l.
7. 12th rib
8. External abdominal oblique m.
9. Internal abdominal oblique m.
10. Transversus abdominis m.
11. Quadratus lumborum m.
12. Psoas minor m.
13. Psoas major m.
14. Iliacus m.
15. Inguinal l.
16. Iliopsoas m.
17. Lesser trochanter of femur
18. Subcostal m.
19. Esophageal hiatus
20. Aortic hiatus
21. Right crus of diaphragm
22. Left crus of diaphragm
23. Thoracolumbar fascia
24. Anterior superior iliac spine
25. Piriformis m.
26. Sacrum
27. Coccygeus m.
28. Coccyx
29. Obturator internus m.
30. Levator ani m.
31. Obturator externus m.

Key: Abbreviations

Ligament—l.
Ligaments—ll.
Muscle—m.
Muscles—mm.
Tendon—t.
Tendons—tt.

Vertebrae:
Cervical—C
Thoracic—T
Lumbar—L

©2008 Wolters Kluwer Health | Lippincott Williams & Wilkins I Published by Anatomical Chart Company, Skokie, IL

The Nervous System

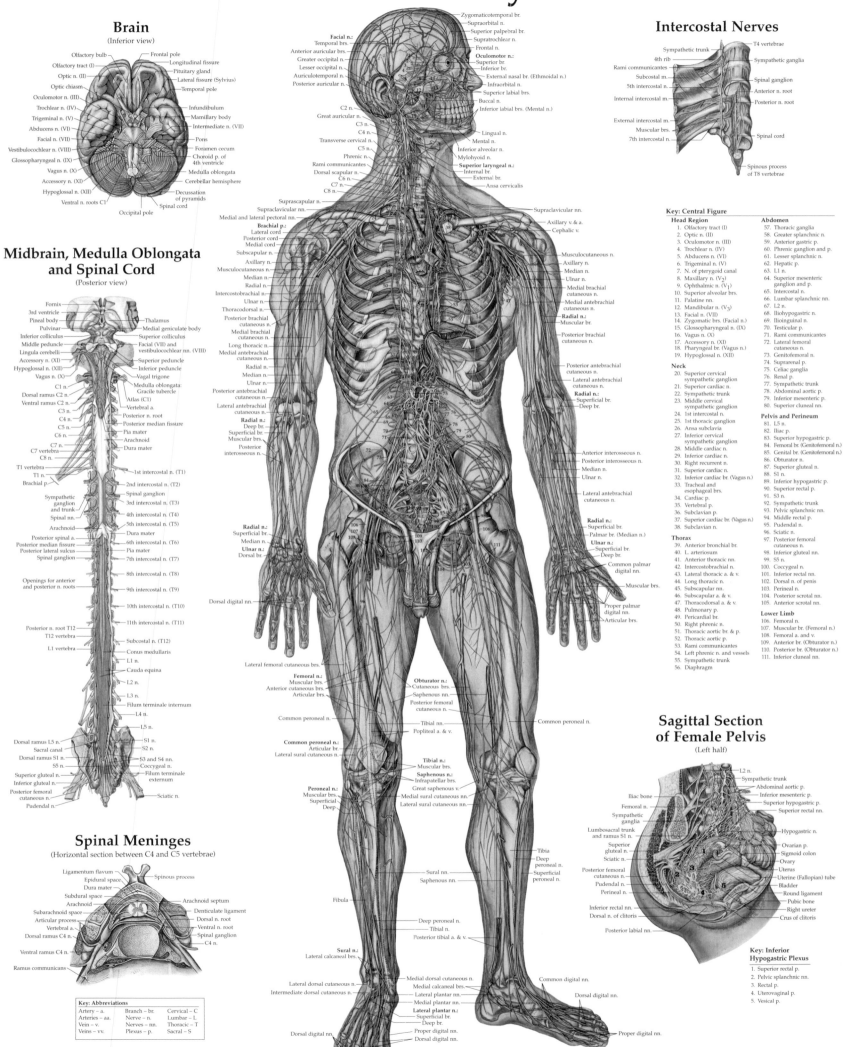

Brain
(Inferior view)

Olfactory bulb
Olfactory tract (I)
Optic n. (II)
Optic chiasm
Oculomotor n. (III)
Trochlear n. (IV)
Trigeminal n. (V)
Abducens n. (VI)
Facial n. (VII)
Vestibulocochlear n. (VIII)
Glossopharyngeal n. (IX)
Vagus n. (X)
Accessory n. (XI)
Hypoglossal n. (XII)
Ventral n. roots C1

Frontal pole
Longitudinal fissure
Pituitary gland
Lateral fissure (Sylvius)
Temporal pole
Infundibulum
Mamillary body
Intermediate n. (VII)
Pons
Foramen cecum
Choroid p. of 4th ventricle
Medulla oblongata
Cerebellar hemisphere
Decussation of pyramids
Spinal cord
Occipital pole

Midbrain, Medulla Oblongata and Spinal Cord
(Posterior view)

Fornix
3rd ventricle
Pineal body
Pulvinar
Inferior colliculus
Middle peduncle
Lingula cerebelli
Accessory n. (XI)
Hypoglossal n. (XII)
Vagus n. (X)

Thalamus
Medial geniculate body
Superior colliculus
Facial (VII) and vestibulocochlear nn. (VIII)
Superior peduncle
Inferior peduncle
Vagal trigone
Medulla oblongata: Gracile tubercle

C1 n.
Dorsal ramus C2 n.
Ventral ramus C2 n.
C3 n.
C4 n.
C5 n.
C6 n.
C7 vertebra
C8 n.
T1 vertebra
T1 n.
Brachial p.

Atlas (C1)
Vertebral a.
Posterior n. root
Posterior median fissure
Pia mater
Arachnoid
Dura mater
1st intercostal n. (T1)
2nd intercostal n. (T2)
Spinal ganglion
3rd intercostal n. (T3)

Sympathetic ganglion and trunk
Spinal nn.
Arachnoid
Posterior spinal a.
Posterior median fissure
Posterior lateral sulcus
Spinal ganglion

4th intercostal n. (T4)
5th intercostal n. (T5)
Dura mater
6th intercostal n. (T6)
Pia mater
7th intercostal n. (T7)

Openings for anterior and posterior n. roots
8th intercostal n. (T8)
9th intercostal n. (T9)
10th intercostal n. (T10)
11th intercostal n. (T11)

Posterior n. root T12
T12 vertebra
L1 vertebra
Subcostal n. (T12)
Conus medullaris
L1 n.
Cauda equina
L2 n.
L3 n.
Filum terminale internum
L4 n.
L5 n.
Dorsal ramus L5 n.
S1 n.
Sacral canal
S2 n.
Dorsal ramus S1 n.
S3 and S4 nn.
S5 n.
Coccygeal n.
Superior gluteal n.
Filum terminale externum
Inferior gluteal n.
Posterior femoral cutaneous n.
Pudendal n.
Sciatic n.

Spinal Meninges
(Horizontal section between C4 and C5 vertebrae)

Ligamentum flavum
Epidural space
Dura mater
Subdural space
Arachnoid
Subarachnoid space
Articular process
Vertebral a.
Dorsal ramus C4 n.
Ventral ramus C4 n.
Ramus communicans

Spinous process
Arachnoid septum
Denticulate ligament
Dorsal n. root
Ventral n. root
Spinal ganglion
C4 n.

Key: Abbreviations

Artery – a.	Branch – br.	Cervical – C
Arteries – aa.	Nerve – n.	Lumbar – L
Vein – v.	Nerves – nn.	Thoracic – T
Veins – vv.	Plexus – p.	Sacral – S

Intercostal Nerves

Sympathetic trunk
4th rib
Rami communicantes
Subcostal m.
5th intercostal n.
Internal intercostal m.
External intercostal m.
Muscular brs.
7th intercostal n.

T4 vertebrae
Sympathetic ganglia
Spinal ganglion
Anterior n. root
Posterior n. root
Spinal cord
Spinous process of T8 vertebrae

Key: Central Figure

Head Region
1. Olfactory tract (I)
2. Optic n. (II)
3. Oculomotor n. (III)
4. Trochlear n. (IV)
5. Abducens n. (VI)
6. Trigeminal n. (V)
7. N. of pterygoid canal
8. Maxillary n. (V_2)
9. Ophthalmic n. (V_1)
10. Superior alveolar brs.
11. Palatine nn.
12. Mandibular n. (V_3)
13. Facial n. (VII)
14. Zygomatic brs. (Facial n.)
15. Glossopharyngeal n. (IX)
16. Vagus n. (X)
17. Accessory n. (XI)
18. Pharyngeal br. (Vagus n.)
19. Hypoglossal n. (XII)

Neck
20. Superior cervical sympathetic ganglion
21. Superior cardiac n.
22. Sympathetic trunk
23. Middle cervical sympathetic ganglion
24. 1st intercostal n.
25. 1st thoracic ganglion
26. Ansa subclavia
27. Inferior cervical sympathetic ganglion
28. Middle cardiac n.
29. Inferior cardiac n.
30. Right recurrent n.
31. Superior cardiac n.
32. Inferior cardiac br. (Vagus n.)
33. Tracheal and esophageal brs.
34. Cardiac p.
35. Vertebral p.
36. Subclavian p.
37. Superior cardiac br. (Vagus n.)
38. Subclavian p.

Thorax
39. Anterior bronchial br.
40. L. arteriosum
41. Anterior thoracic nn.
42. Intercostobrachial n.
43. Lateral thoracic a. & v.
44. Long thoracic n.
45. Subscapular nn.
46. Subscapular a. & v.
47. Thoracodorsal a. & v.
48. Pulmonary p.
49. Pericardial br.
50. Right phrenic n.
51. Thoracic aortic br. & p.
52. Thoracic aortic p.
53. Rami communicantes
54. Left phrenic n. and vessels
55. Sympathetic trunk
56. Diaphragm

Abdomen
57. Thoracic ganglia
58. Greater splanchnic n.
59. Anterior gastric p.
60. Phrenic ganglion and p.
61. Lesser splanchnic n.
62. Hepatic p.
63. L1 n.
64. Superior mesenteric ganglion and p.
65. Intercostal n.
66. Lumbar splanchnic nn.
67. L2 n.
68. Iliohypogastric n.
69. Ilioinguinal n.
70. Testicular p.
71. Rami communicantes
72. Lateral femoral cutaneous n.
73. Genitofemoral n.
74. Suprarenal p.
75. Celiac ganglia
76. Renal p.
77. Sympathetic trunk
78. Abdominal aortic p.
79. Inferior mesenteric p.
80. Superior cluneal nn.

Pelvis and Perineum
81. L5 n.
82. Iliac p.
83. Superior hypogastric p.
84. Femoral br. (Genitofemoral n.)
85. Genital br. (Genitofemoral n.)
86. Obturator n.
87. Superior gluteal n.
88. S1 n.
89. Inferior hypogastric p.
90. Superior rectal p.
91. S3 n.
92. Sympathetic trunk
93. Pelvic splanchnic nn.
94. Middle rectal p.
95. Pudendal n.
96. Sciatic n.
97. Posterior femoral cutaneous n.
98. Inferior gluteal nn.
99. S5 n.
100. Coccygeal n.
101. Inferior rectal nn.
102. Dorsal n. of penis
103. Perineal n.
104. Posterior scrotal nn.
105. Anterior scrotal nn.

Lower Limb
106. Femoral n.
107. Muscular br. (Femoral n.)
108. Femoral a. and v.
109. Anterior br. (Obturator n.)
110. Posterior br. (Obturator n.)
111. Inferior cluneal nn.

Central figure labels

Zygomaticotemporal br.
Supraorbital n.
Superior palpebral br.
Supratrochlear n.
Frontal n.
Oculomotor n.:
Superior br.
Inferior br.
External nasal br. (Ethmoidal n.)
Infraorbital n.
Superior labial brs.
Buccal n.
Inferior labial brs. (Mental n.)
Lingual n.
Mental n.
Inferior alveolar n.
Mylohyoid n.

Facial n.:
Temporal brs.
Anterior auricular brs.
Greater occipital n.
Lesser occipital n.
Auriculotemporal n.
Posterior auricular n.

C2 n.
Great auricular n.
C3 n.
C4 n.
Transverse cervical n.
C5 n.
Phrenic n.
Rami communicantes
Dorsal scapular n.
C6 n.
C7 n.
C8 n.

Superior laryngeal n.:
Internal br.
External br.
Ansa cervicalis

Suprascapular n.
Supraclavicular n.
Medial and lateral pectoral nn.
Brachial p.:
Lateral cord
Posterior cord
Medial cord
Subscapular n.
Axillary n.
Musculocutaneous n.
Median n.
Radial n.
Intercostobrachial n.
Thoracodorsal n.
Posterior brachial cutaneous n.
Medial brachial cutaneous n.
Long thoracic n.
Medial antebrachial cutaneous n.
Radial n.
Median n.
Ulnar n.
Posterior antebrachial cutaneous n.
Lateral antebrachial cutaneous n.
Radial n.:
Deep br.
Superficial br.
Muscular br.
Posterior interosseous n.

Supraclavicular nn.
Axillary v. & a.
Cephalic v.
Musculocutaneous n.
Axillary n.
Median n.
Ulnar n.
Medial brachial cutaneous n.
Medial antebrachial cutaneous n.
Radial n.:
Muscular br.
Posterior brachial cutaneous n.
Posterior antebrachial cutaneous n.
Lateral antebrachial cutaneous n.
Radial n.:
Superficial br.
Deep br.

Anterior interosseous n.
Posterior interosseous n.
Median n.
Ulnar n.
Lateral antebrachial cutaneous n.
Radial n.:
Superficial br.
Ulnar n.:
Superficial br.
Deep br.
Common palmar digital nn.
Muscular brs.
Proper palmar digital nn.
Articular brs.

Radial n.:
Superficial br.
Median n.
Ulnar n.:
Dorsal br.
Dorsal digital nn.

Lateral femoral cutaneous brs.
Femoral n.:
Muscular brs.
Anterior cutaneous brs.
Articular brs.
Common peroneal n.

Common peroneal n.:
Articular br.
Lateral sural cutaneous n.
Peroneal n.:
Muscular brs.
Superficial
Deep
Fibula

Obturator n.:
Cutaneous brs.
Saphenous nn.
Posterior femoral cutaneous n.
Tibial nn.
Popliteal a. & v.
Common peroneal n.

Tibial n.:
Muscular brs.
Saphenous n.:
Infrapatellar brs.
Great saphenous v.
Medial sural cutaneous nn.
Lateral sural cutaneous n.

Tibia
Deep peroneal n.
Superficial peroneal n.
Sural nn.
Saphenous nn.

Deep peroneal n.
Tibial n.
Posterior tibial a. & v.
Posterior labial nn.

Sural n.:
Lateral calcaneal brs.

Lateral dorsal cutaneous n.
Intermediate dorsal cutaneous n.
Medial dorsal cutaneous n.
Medial calcaneal brs.
Lateral plantar nn.
Medial plantar nn.
Lateral plantar n.:
Superficial br.
Deep br.
Common digital nn.
Dorsal digital nn.
Dorsal digital nn.
Proper digital nn.
Proper digital nn.

Sagittal Section of Female Pelvis
(Left half)

Iliac bone
Femoral n.
Sympathetic ganglia
Lumbosacral trunk and ramus S1 n.
Superior gluteal n.
Sciatic n.
Posterior femoral cutaneous n.
Pudendal n.
Perineal n.
Inferior rectal nn.
Dorsal n. of clitoris
Posterior labial nn.

L2 n.
Sympathetic trunk
Abdominal aortic p.
Inferior mesenteric p.
Superior hypogastric p.
Superior rectal nn.
Hypogastric n.
Ovarian p.
Sigmoid colon
Ovary
Uterus
Uterine (Fallopian) tube
Bladder
Round ligament
Pubic bone
Right ureter
Crus of clitoris

Key: Inferior Hypogastric Plexus
1. Superior rectal p.
2. Pelvic splanchnic nn.
3. Rectal p.
4. Uterovaginal p.
5. Vesical p.

©2008 Wolters Kluwer Health | Lippincott Williams & Wilkins | Published by Anatomical Chart Company, Skokie, IL

The Respiratory System

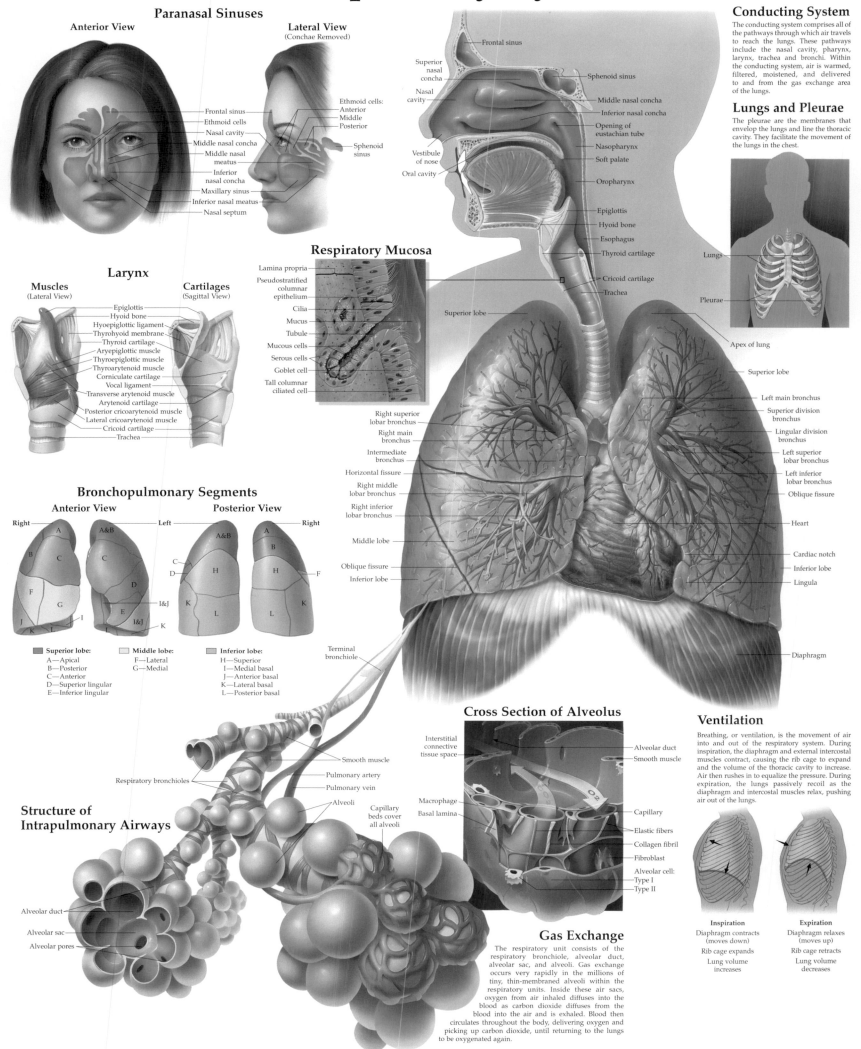

Paranasal Sinuses

Anterior View

- Frontal sinus
- Ethmoid cells
- Nasal cavity
- Middle nasal concha
- Middle nasal meatus
- Inferior nasal concha
- Maxillary sinus
- Inferior nasal meatus
- Nasal septum

Lateral View
(Conchae Removed)

- Ethmoid cells:
  - Anterior
  - Middle
  - Posterior
- Sphenoid sinus

Larynx

Muscles
(Lateral View)

Cartilages
(Sagittal View)

- Epiglottis
- Hyoid bone
- Hyoepiglottic ligament
- Thyrohyoid membrane
- Thyroid cartilage
- Aryepiglottic muscle
- Thyroepiglottic muscle
- Thyroarytenoid muscle
- Corniculate cartilage
- Vocal ligament
- Transverse arytenoid muscle
- Arytenoid cartilage
- Posterior cricoarytenoid muscle
- Lateral cricoarytenoid muscle
- Cricoid cartilage
- Trachea

Respiratory Mucosa

- Lamina propria
- Pseudostratified columnar epithelium
- Cilia
- Mucus
- Tubule
- Mucous cells
- Serous cells
- Goblet cell
- Tall columnar ciliated cell

Bronchopulmonary Segments

Anterior View

Right — Left

Posterior View

Left — Right

- A&B
- A
- B
- C
- D
- E
- F
- G
- H
- I
- I&J
- J
- K
- L

Superior lobe:
- A—Apical
- B—Posterior
- C—Anterior
- D—Superior lingular
- E—Inferior lingular

Middle lobe:
- F—Lateral
- G—Medial

Inferior lobe:
- H—Superior
- I—Medial basal
- J—Anterior basal
- K—Lateral basal
- L—Posterior basal

Central figure labels:

- Frontal sinus
- Superior nasal concha
- Nasal cavity
- Vestibule of nose
- Oral cavity
- Sphenoid sinus
- Middle nasal concha
- Inferior nasal concha
- Opening of eustachian tube
- Nasopharynx
- Soft palate
- Oropharynx
- Epiglottis
- Hyoid bone
- Esophagus
- Thyroid cartilage
- Cricoid cartilage
- Trachea
- Superior lobe
- Right superior lobar bronchus
- Right main bronchus
- Intermediate bronchus
- Horizontal fissure
- Right middle lobar bronchus
- Right inferior lobar bronchus
- Middle lobe
- Oblique fissure
- Inferior lobe
- Left main bronchus
- Superior division bronchus
- Lingular division bronchus
- Left superior lobar bronchus
- Left inferior lobar bronchus
- Oblique fissure
- Heart
- Cardiac notch
- Inferior lobe
- Lingula
- Diaphragm

Conducting System

The conducting system comprises all of the pathways through which air travels to reach the lungs. These pathways include the nasal cavity, pharynx, larynx, trachea and bronchi. Within the conducting system, air is warmed, filtered, moistened, and delivered to and from the gas exchange area of the lungs.

Lungs and Pleurae

The pleurae are the membranes that envelop the lungs and line the thoracic cavity. They facilitate the movement of the lungs in the chest.

- Lungs
- Pleurae
- Apex of lung

Structure of Intrapulmonary Airways

- Terminal bronchiole
- Smooth muscle
- Pulmonary artery
- Pulmonary vein
- Alveoli
- Capillary beds cover all alveoli
- Respiratory bronchioles
- Alveolar duct
- Alveolar sac
- Alveolar pores

Cross Section of Alveolus

- Interstitial connective tissue space
- Macrophage
- Basal lamina
- Alveolar duct
- Smooth muscle
- Capillary
- Elastic fibers
- Collagen fibril
- Fibroblast
- Alveolar cell:
  - Type I
  - Type II

Gas Exchange

The respiratory unit consists of the respiratory bronchiole, alveolar duct, alveolar sac, and alveoli. Gas exchange occurs very rapidly in the millions of tiny, thin-membraned alveoli within the respiratory units. Inside these air sacs, oxygen from air inhaled diffuses into the blood as carbon dioxide diffuses from the blood into the air and is exhaled. Blood then circulates throughout the body, delivering oxygen and picking up carbon dioxide, until returning to the lungs to be oxygenated again.

Ventilation

Breathing, or ventilation, is the movement of air into and out of the respiratory system. During inspiration, the diaphragm and external intercostal muscles contract, causing the rib cage to expand and the volume of the thoracic cavity to increase. Air then rushes in to equalize the pressure. During expiration, the lungs passively recoil as the diaphragm and intercostal muscles relax, pushing air out of the lungs.

Inspiration
Diaphragm contracts (moves down)
Rib cage expands
Lung volume increases

Expiration
Diaphragm relaxes (moves up)
Rib cage retracts
Lung volume decreases

©2008 Wolters Kluwer Health | Lippincott Williams & Wilkins I Published by Anatomical Chart Company, Skokie, IL

The Skeletal System

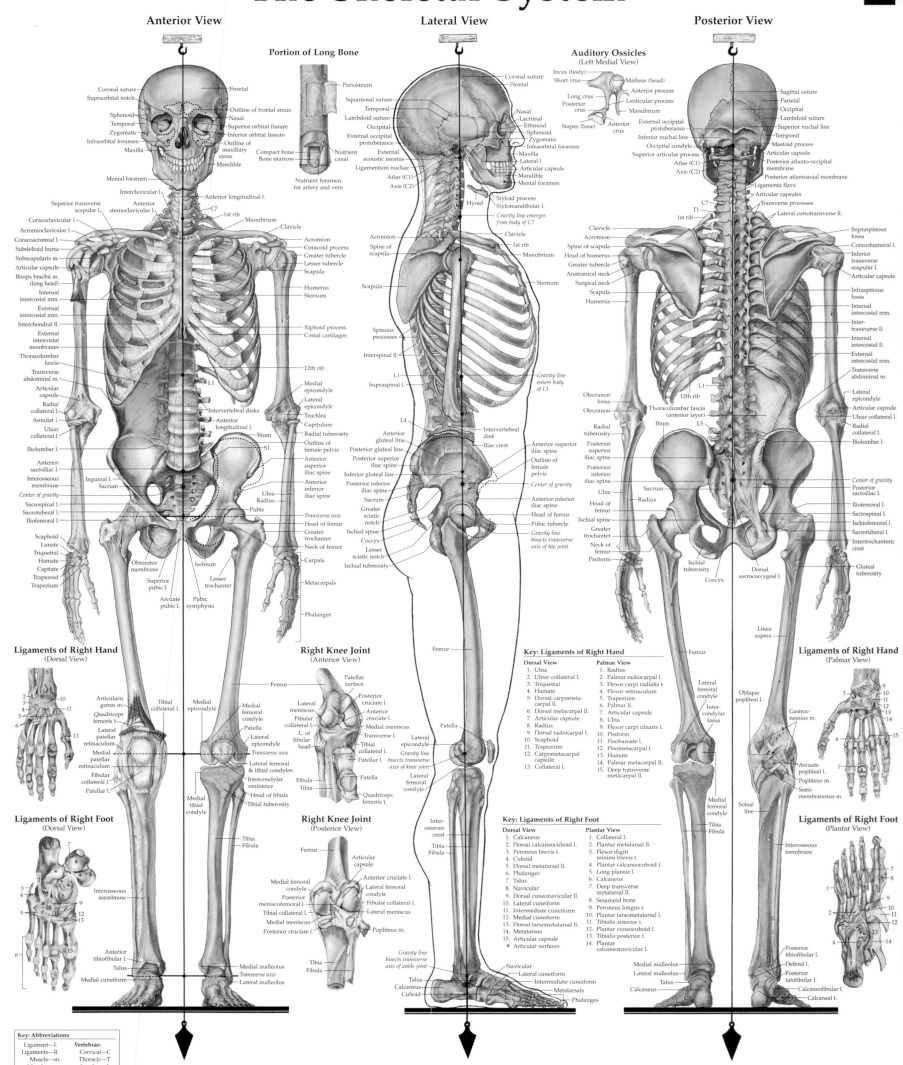

The Spinal Nerves

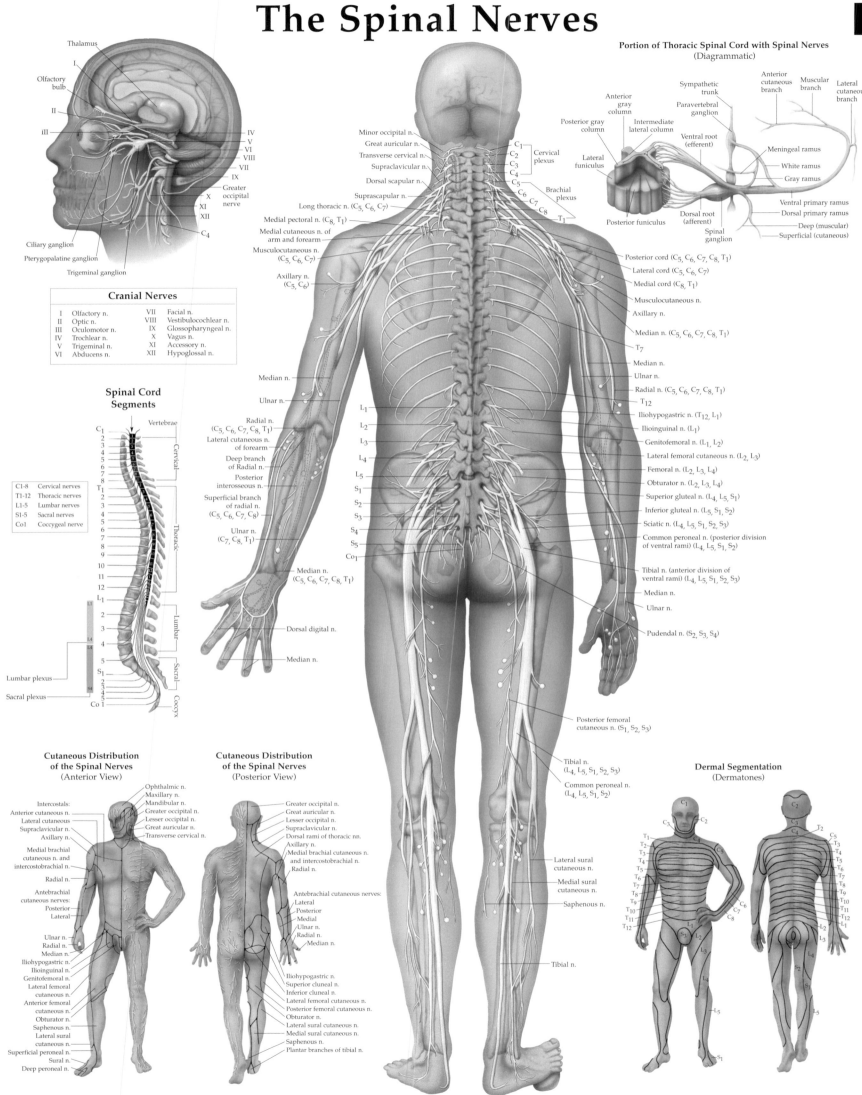

Cranial Nerves

I	Olfactory n.	VII	Facial n.
II	Optic n.	VIII	Vestibulocochlear n.
III	Oculomotor n.	IX	Glossopharyngeal n.
IV	Trochlear n.	X	Vagus n.
V	Trigeminal n.	XI	Accessory n.
VI	Abducens n.	XII	Hypoglossal n.

Spinal Cord Segments

C1-8	Cervical nerves
T1-12	Thoracic nerves
L1-5	Lumbar nerves
S1-5	Sacral nerves
Co1	Coccygeal nerve

Portion of Thoracic Spinal Cord with Spinal Nerves
(Diagrammatic)

Cutaneous Distribution of the Spinal Nerves
(Anterior View)

Cutaneous Distribution of the Spinal Nerves
(Posterior View)

Dermal Segmentation
(Dermatones)

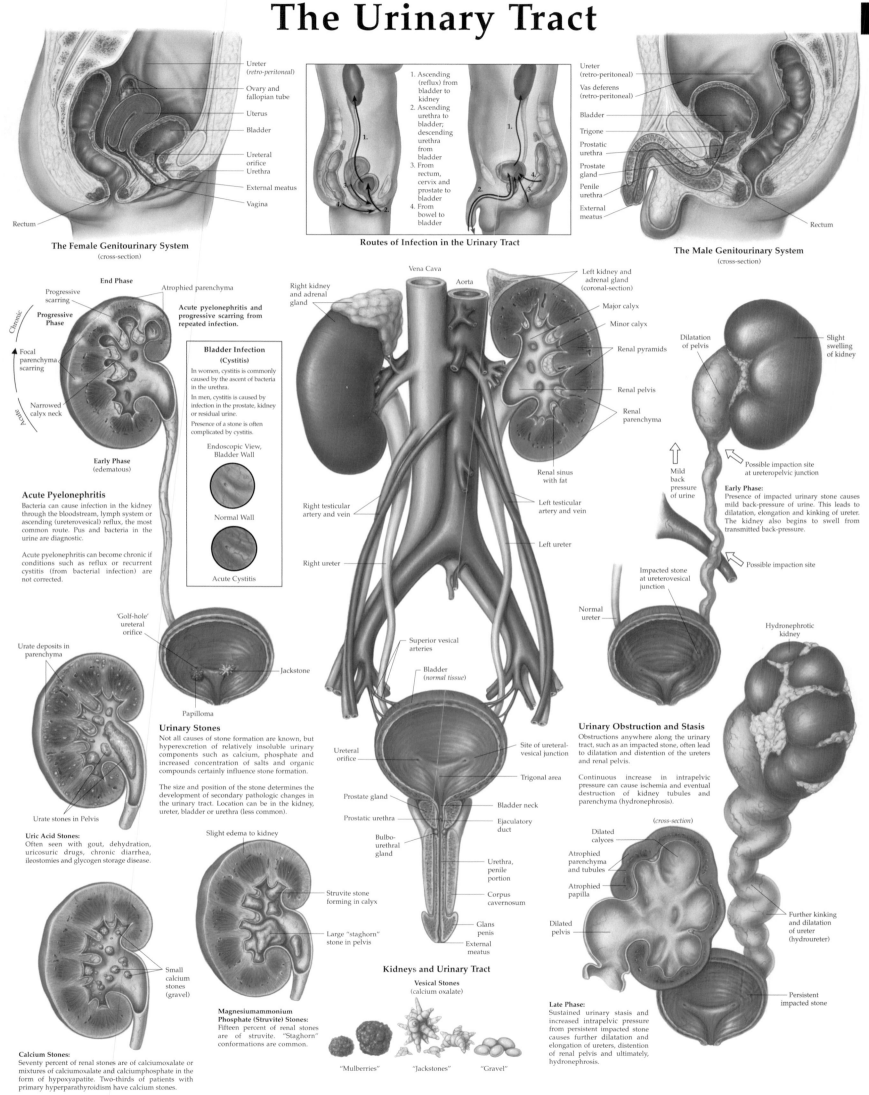

The Female Genitourinary System
(cross-section)

- Ureter (retro-peritoneal)
- Ovary and fallopian tube
- Uterus
- Bladder
- Ureteral orifice
- Urethra
- External meatus
- Vagina
- Rectum

Routes of Infection in the Urinary Tract

1. Ascending (reflux) from bladder to kidney
2. Ascending urethra to bladder; descending urethra from bladder
3. From rectum, cervix and prostate to bladder
4. From bowel to bladder

The Male Genitourinary System
(cross-section)

- Ureter (retro-peritoneal)
- Vas deferens (retro-peritoneal)
- Bladder
- Trigone
- Prostatic urethra
- Prostate gland
- Penile urethra
- External meatus
- Rectum

End Phase
Progressive scarring
Atrophied parenchyma
Progressive Phase
Focal parenchyma scarring
Narrowed calyx neck
Early Phase (edematous)

Acute pyelonephritis and progressive scarring from repeated infection.

Acute Pyelonephritis
Bacteria can cause infection in the kidney through the bloodstream, lymph system or ascending (ureterovesical) reflux, the most common route. Pus and bacteria in the urine are diagnostic.

Acute pyelonephritis can become chronic if conditions such as reflux or recurrent cystitis (from bacterial infection) are not corrected.

Bladder Infection (Cystitis)
In women, cystitis is commonly caused by the ascent of bacteria in the urethra.
In men, cystitis is caused by infection in the prostate, kidney or residual urine.
Presence of a stone is often complicated by cystitis.

Endoscopic View, Bladder Wall
Normal Wall
Acute Cystitis

'Golf-hole' ureteral orifice
Papilloma
Jackstone

Urate deposits in parenchyma
Urate stones in Pelvis

Urinary Stones
Not all causes of stone formation are known, but hyperexcretion of relatively insoluble urinary components such as calcium, phosphate and increased concentration of salts and organic compounds certainly influence stone formation.

The size and position of the stone determines the development of secondary pathologic changes in the urinary tract. Location can be in the kidney, ureter, bladder or urethra (less common).

Uric Acid Stones:
Often seen with gout, dehydration, uricosuric drugs, chronic diarrhea, ileostomies and glycogen storage disease.

Slight edema to kidney
Struvite stone forming in calyx
Large "staghorn" stone in pelvis
Small calcium stones (gravel)

Magnesiumammonium Phosphate (Struvite) Stones:
Fifteen percent of renal stones are of struvite. "Staghorn" conformations are common.

Calcium Stones:
Seventy percent of renal stones are of calciumoxalate or mixtures of calciumoxalate and calciumphosphate in the form of hypoxyapatite. Two-thirds of patients with primary hyperparathyroidism have calcium stones.

Vena Cava
Aorta
Right kidney and adrenal gland
Left kidney and adrenal gland (coronal-section)
Major calyx
Minor calyx
Renal pyramids
Renal pelvis
Renal parenchyma
Renal sinus with fat
Right testicular artery and vein
Left testicular artery and vein
Left ureter
Right ureter
Superior vesical arteries
Bladder (normal tissue)
Ureteral orifice
Site of ureteral-vesical junction
Trigonal area
Prostate gland
Bladder neck
Prostatic urethra
Ejaculatory duct
Bulbo-urethral gland
Urethra, penile portion
Corpus cavernosum
Glans penis
External meatus

Kidneys and Urinary Tract

Vesical Stones (calcium oxalate)
"Mulberries"   "Jackstones"   "Gravel"

Dilatation of pelvis
Slight swelling of kidney
Mild back pressure of urine
Possible impaction site at ureteropelvic junction

Early Phase:
Presence of impacted urinary stone causes mild back-pressure of urine. This leads to dilatation, elongation and kinking of ureter. The kidney also begins to swell from transmitted back-pressure.

Possible impaction site
Impacted stone at ureterovesical junction
Normal ureter
Hydronephrotic kidney

Urinary Obstruction and Stasis
Obstructions anywhere along the urinary tract, such as an impacted stone, often lead to dilatation and distention of the ureters and renal pelvis.

Continuous increase in intrapelvic pressure can cause ischemia and eventual destruction of kidney tubules and parenchyma (hydronephrosis).

(cross-section)
Dilated calyces
Atrophied parenchyma and tubules
Atrophied papilla
Dilated pelvis
Further kinking and dilatation of ureter (hydroureter)
Persistent impacted stone

Late Phase:
Sustained urinary stasis and increased intrapelvic pressure from persistent impacted stone causes further dilatation and elongation of ureters, distention of renal pelvis and ultimately, hydronephrosis.

©2008 Wolters Kluwer Health | Lippincott Williams & Wilkins | Published by Anatomical Chart Company, Skokie, IL

The Vascular System and Viscera

Heart (Right interior view)

Heart (Left interior view)

Heart (Posterior view)

Heart in Systole
(Superior view, atria removed)

Female Pelvis
(Posterior view)

Base of the Brain
(Left cerebellum removed)

Key: Central Figure

1. Parietal pleura
2. Right internal thoracic a. & v.
3. Right brachiocephalic v.
4. Brachiocephalic trunk
5. Left common carotid a.
6. Superior vena cava
7. Pericardium
8. Ascending aorta
9. Pulmonary trunk
10. Left pulmonary a.
11. Right lung
12. Right atrium and auricle
13. Left auricle
14. Left pulmonary vv.
15. Right coronary a.
16. Anterior interventricular a.
17. Diaphragm
18. Hepatic vv.
19. Inferior vena cava
20. Inferior phrenic aa.
21. Superior suprarenal aa.
22. Right suprarenal gland
23. Middle and inferior suprarenal aa.
24. Right kidney
25. Testicular aa. & vv.
26. 10th rib
27. Abdominal aorta
28. Inferior mesenteric a.
29. Ascending lumbar v.
30. Common iliac aa. & vv.
31. Anterior superior iliac spine
32. Iliacus muscle
33. Iliolumbar a. & v.
34. Internal iliac a. & v.
35. Deep circumflex iliac a.
36. Superior vesicle a.
37. Urinary bladder
38. Cremasteric a.
39. Obturator a.
40. Spermatic cord
41. Esophagus
42. Spleen
43. Aortic hiatus
44. Celiac trunk
45. Superior mesenteric a.
46. Left renal a. & v.
47. Ureter
48. Quadratus lumborum muscle
49. 4th lumbar a. & v.
50. Middle sacral a.
51. Superior gluteal a. & v.
52. External iliac a. & v.
53. Inguinal ligament
54. Inferior epigastric a.
55. Superficial circumflex iliac a. & v.
56. External pudendal aa. & vv.
57. Internal pudendal a. & vv.
58. Deep dorsal v. and dorsal a. of penis
59. Pampiniform venous plexus
60. Testicle

Branches of Abdominal Aorta and Portal Vein

Key: Vessels of Abdomen

1. Intercostal a. & v.
2. Azygos v.
3. Thoracic duct
4. Thoracic aorta
5. Hemiazygos v.
6. Esophageal venous plexus
7. Hepatic v.
8. Inferior vena cava
9. Common hepatic duct
10. Proper hepatic a.
11. Cystic duct
12. Common bile duct
13. Gastroduodenal a.
14. Anterior superior pancreaticoduodenal a. & v.
15. Pancreatic duct
16. Anterior inferior pancreaticoduodenal a. & v.
17. Right colic a.
18. Ileocolic a.
19. Left gastric a.
20. Short gastric aa. & vv.
21. Inferior phrenic a.
22. Celiac trunk
23. Common hepatic a.
24. Splenic a.
25. Cisterna chyli
26. Right gastric a.
27. Portal v.
28. Left gastroepiploic a. & v.
29. Superior mesenteric a.
30. Right gastroepiploic a. & v.
31. Middle colic a. & v.
32. Jejunal & ileal aa. & vv.
33. Inferior mesenteric a.
34. Left colic a. & v.
35. Common iliac aa. & vv.
36. Sigmoid aa. & vv.
37. Middle sacral a. & v.
38. Superior rectal a. & v.
39. Right internal iliac a. & v.
40. Middle rectal a. & v.
41. Inferior rectal a. & v.

Key: Abbreviations

Artery – a.	Cervical vertebra – C
Arteries – aa.	Nerve – n.
Branch – br.	Vein – v.
Branches – brs.	Veins – vv.

©2008 Wolters Kluwer Health | Lippincott Williams & Wilkins | Published by Anatomical Chart Company, Skokie, IL

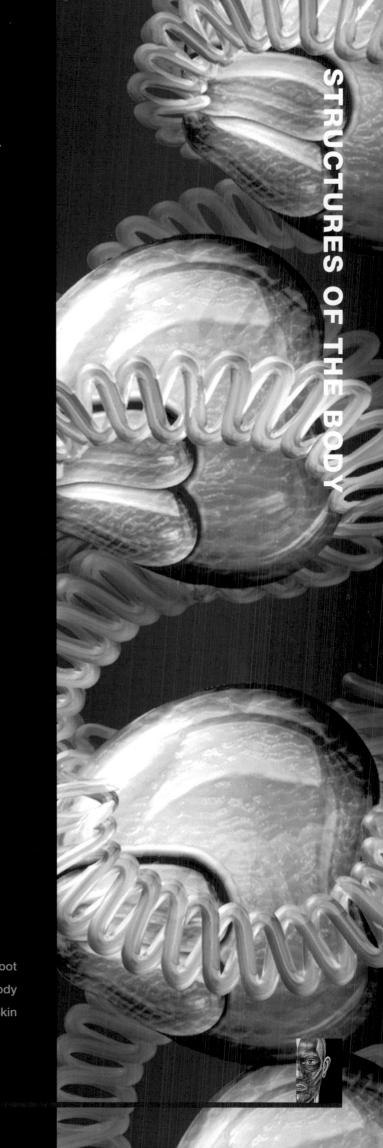

STRUCTURES OF THE BODY

The Brain

Arteries of the Brain
(Lateral View)

- Central a.
- Precentral a.
- Ascending frontal a.
- Lateral orbito-frontal a.
- Middle cerebral a.
- Anterior temporal a.
- Middle temporal a.
- Basilar a.
- Internal carotid a.
- Anterior spinal a.
- Anterior parietal a.
- Posterior parietal a.
- Angular a.
- Posterior temporal a.
- Anterior inferior cerebellar a.
- Posterior inferior cerebellar a.
- Vertebral a.

Base of Brain
(Cranial Nerves)

- Eyeball
- Olfactory bulb
- Optic n. (II)
- Olfactory tract (I)
- Optic chiasm
- Lateral olfactory stria
- Trigeminal n. (V):
  - Ophthalmic n. (V₁)
  - Maxillary n. (V₂)
  - Mandibular n. (V₃)
- Trigeminal ganglion
- Pons
- Hypoglossal n. (XII)
- Vagus n. (X)
- Accessory n. (XI)
- Optic tract
- Oculomotor n. (III)
- Trochlear n. (IV)
- Abducens n. (VI)
- Facial n. (VII)
- Vestibulocochlear n. (VIII)
- Glossopharyngeal n. (IX)
- Medulla oblongata
- Ventral root of 1st spinal n.
- Spinal cord

Lobes of the Brain

- Cerebrum
- Cerebellum

Key
- Frontal lobe
- Parietal lobe
- Temporal lobe
- Occipital lobe

Limbic System

- Cingulate gyrus
- Corpus callosum
- Body of fornix
- Stria medullaris thalami
- Stria terminalis
- Mamillary body
- Olfactory tract
- Amygdala
- Hippocampus

Arteries of the Brain
(Sagittal Section)

- Medial frontal branches:
  - Posterior
  - Middle
  - Anterior
- Calloso-marginal a.
- Frontopolar a.
- Anterior cerebral a.
- Medial orbitofrontal a.
- Internal carotid a.
- Pituitary gland
- Posterior communicating a.
- Paracentral a.
- Precuneal a.
- Corpus callosum
- Posterior pericallosal a.
- Parieto-occipital a.
- Pineal body
- Calcarine a.
- Posterior cerebral a.

Base of Brain
(Vessels)

- Medial orbitofrontal a.
- Anterior communicating a.
- Middle cerebral a.
- Internal carotid a.
- Posterior communicating a.
- Posterior cerebral a.
- Anterior cerebral a.
- Superior cerebellar a.
- Pontine aa.
- Basilar a.
- Internal acoustic a.
- Anterior inferior cerebellar a.
- Vertebral a.
- Anterior spinal a.
- Posterior spinal a.
- Transverse sinus

Axial view

Ventricles of the Brain
(Lateral View)

Key

A. Lateral ventricle:
  1. Anterior horn
  2. Posterior horn
  3. Inferior horn
B. Interventricular foramen (Monro)
C. Third ventricle
D. Cerebral aqueduct
E. Lateral aperture (Luschka)
F. Fourth ventricle
G. Median aperture (Magendie)

Coronal Section

- Longitudinal cerebral fissure
- White matter
- Corpus callosum
- Caudate nucleus
- Thalamus
- Claustrum
- Hippocampus
- Pons
- Choroid plexus of 4th ventricle
- Medulla oblongata
- Cerebral cortex (gray matter)
- Lateral ventricle
- Lateral sulcus
- Lentiform nucleus
- 3rd ventricle
- Optic tract
- Interpeduncular cistern
- Cerebellum

Circle of Willis

- Anterior communicating a.
- Anterior cerebral a.
- Middle cerebral a.
- Internal carotid a.
- Posterior communicating a.
- Posterior cerebral a.
- Superior cerebellar a.
- Pontine aa.
- Basilar a.
- Internal acoustic a.
- Anterior inferior cerebellar a.
- Vertebral a.
- Posterior spinal a.
- Anterior spinal a.

Circulation of Cerebrospinal Fluid (CSF)

Choroid plexuses located in the lateral (A), third (B), and fourth (C) ventricles constantly produce CSF. The fluid circulates through the ventricles and foramina of the brain and within the subarachnoid space surrounding the brain and spinal cord. CSF drains into the venous blood by passing through arachnoid granulations located in the dura mater just above the brain (D). Arrows in the adjacent illustration demonstrate the flow of CSF.

Somatotopic Organization of the Cerebrum

Motor Activity*

Sensory Activity*

- Cortex
- Hip, Knee, Trunk, Shoulder, Elbow, Wrist, Hand, Fingers, Thumb, Neck, Brow, Eyelid, Nose, Lips, Jaw
- Elbow, Shoulder, Hip, Knee, Leg, Ankle, Toes
- Wrist, Finger, Thumb, Neck, Brow, Eyelid, Nose, Lips, Tongue, Larynx

- Primary motor area
- Precentral gyrus
- Secondary motor area
- Broca's motor speech area
- Primary auditory area
- Secondary auditory area
- Primary somatosensory area
- Secondary somatosensory area
- Central sulcus
- Secondary visual areas
- Primary visual area

*The exaggerated caricatures sprawling over the illustrations above represent approximate centers within the brain for sensory and motor activities of the named body parts.

Meninges of the Brain

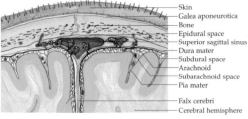

- Skin
- Galea aponeurotica
- Bone
- Epidural space
- Superior sagittal sinus
- Dura mater
- Subdural space
- Arachnoid
- Subarachnoid space
- Pia mater
- Falx cerebri
- Cerebral hemisphere

Key: Abbreviations
- Artery—a.
- Arteries—aa.
- Nerve—n.

©2008 Wolters Kluwer Health | Lippincott Williams & Wilkins | Published by Anatomical Chart Company, Skokie, IL

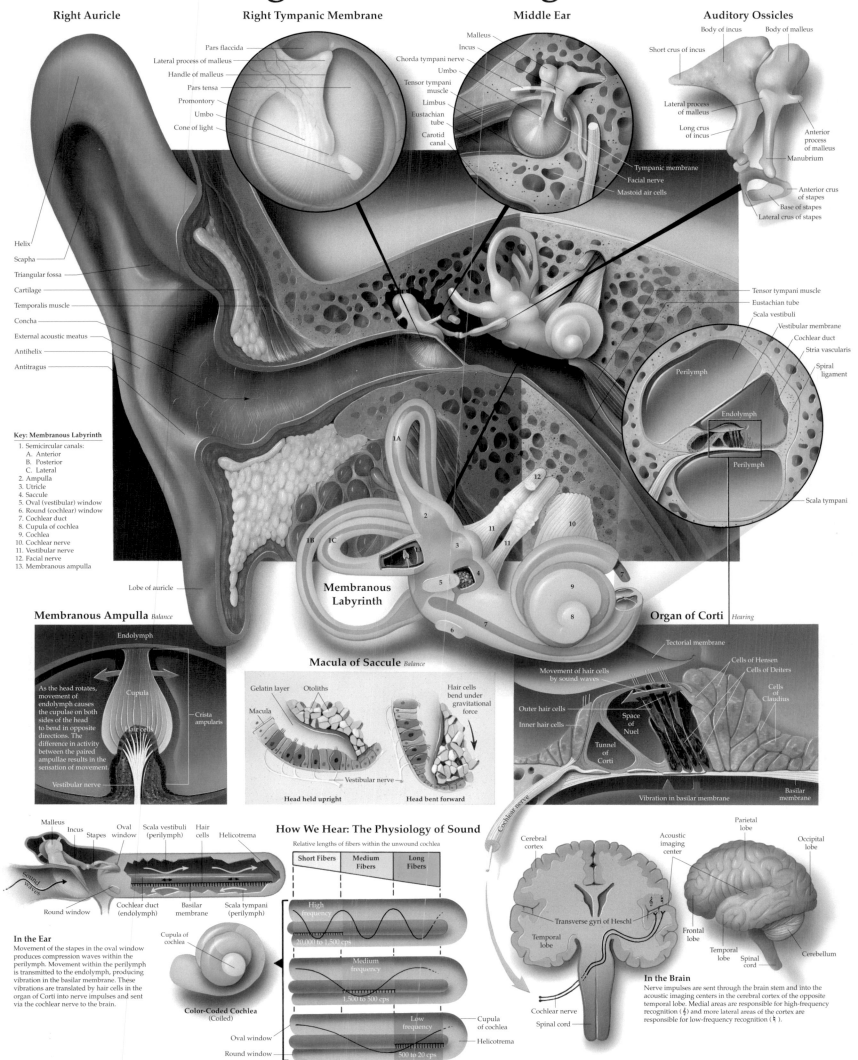

Right Auricle

Right Tympanic Membrane

Pars flaccida
Lateral process of malleus
Handle of malleus
Pars tensa
Promontory
Umbo
Cone of light

Middle Ear

Malleus
Incus
Chorda tympani nerve
Umbo
Tensor tympani muscle
Limbus
Eustachian tube
Carotid canal
Tympanic membrane
Facial nerve
Mastoid air cells

Auditory Ossicles

Body of incus
Body of malleus
Short crus of incus
Lateral process of malleus
Long crus of incus
Anterior process of malleus
Manubrium
Anterior crus of stapes
Base of stapes
Lateral crus of stapes

Helix
Scapha
Triangular fossa
Cartilage
Temporalis muscle
Concha
External acoustic meatus
Antihelix
Antitragus

Tensor tympani muscle
Eustachian tube
Scala vestibuli
Vestibular membrane
Cochlear duct
Stria vascularis
Spiral ligament
Perilymph
Endolymph
Perilymph
Scala tympani

Key: Membranous Labyrinth
1. Semicircular canals:
   A. Anterior
   B. Posterior
   C. Lateral
2. Ampulla
3. Utricle
4. Saccule
5. Oval (vestibular) window
6. Round (cochlear) window
7. Cochlear duct
8. Cupula of cochlea
9. Cochlea
10. Cochlear nerve
11. Vestibular nerve
12. Facial nerve
13. Membranous ampulla

Lobe of auricle

Membranous Labyrinth

Membranous Ampulla *Balance*

Endolymph
Cupula
Crista ampularis
Hair cells
Vestibular nerve

As the head rotates, movement of endolymph causes the cupulae on both sides of the head to bend in opposite directions. The difference in activity between the paired ampullae results in the sensation of movement.

Macula of Saccule *Balance*

Gelatin layer
Otoliths
Macula
Hair cells bend under gravitational force
Vestibular nerve

Head held upright   **Head bent forward**

Organ of Corti *Hearing*

Tectorial membrane
Movement of hair cells by sound waves
Cells of Hensen
Cells of Deiters
Cells of Claudius
Outer hair cells
Inner hair cells
Space of Nuel
Tunnel of Corti
Cochlear nerve
Vibration in basilar membrane
Basilar membrane

How We Hear: The Physiology of Sound

Malleus
Incus
Stapes
Oval window
Scala vestibuli (perilymph)
Hair cells
Helicotrema
Sound waves
Round window
Cochlear duct (endolymph)
Basilar membrane
Scala tympani (perilymph)

Relative lengths of fibers within the unwound cochlea

Short Fibers	Medium Fibers	Long Fibers

High frequency
20,000 to 1,500 cps

Medium frequency
1,500 to 500 cps

Low frequency
500 to 20 cps

Cupula of cochlea
Color-Coded Cochlea (Coiled)
Oval window
Round window
Cupula of cochlea
Helicotrema

In the Ear
Movement of the stapes in the oval window produces compression waves within the perilymph. Movement within the perilymph is transmitted to the endolymph, producing vibration in the basilar membrane. These vibrations are translated by hair cells in the organ of Corti into nerve impulses and sent via the cochlear nerve to the brain.

Cerebral cortex
Acoustic imaging center
Parietal lobe
Occipital lobe
Transverse gyri of Heschl
Temporal lobe
Frontal lobe
Temporal lobe
Spinal cord
Cerebellum
Cochlear nerve
Spinal cord

In the Brain
Nerve impulses are sent through the brain stem and into the acoustic imaging centers in the cerebral cortex of the opposite temporal lobe. Medial areas are responsible for high-frequency recognition (♪) and more lateral areas of the cortex are responsible for low-frequency recognition (♮).

©2008 Wolters Kluwer Health | Lippincott Williams & Wilkins | Published by Anatomical Chart Company, Skokie, IL

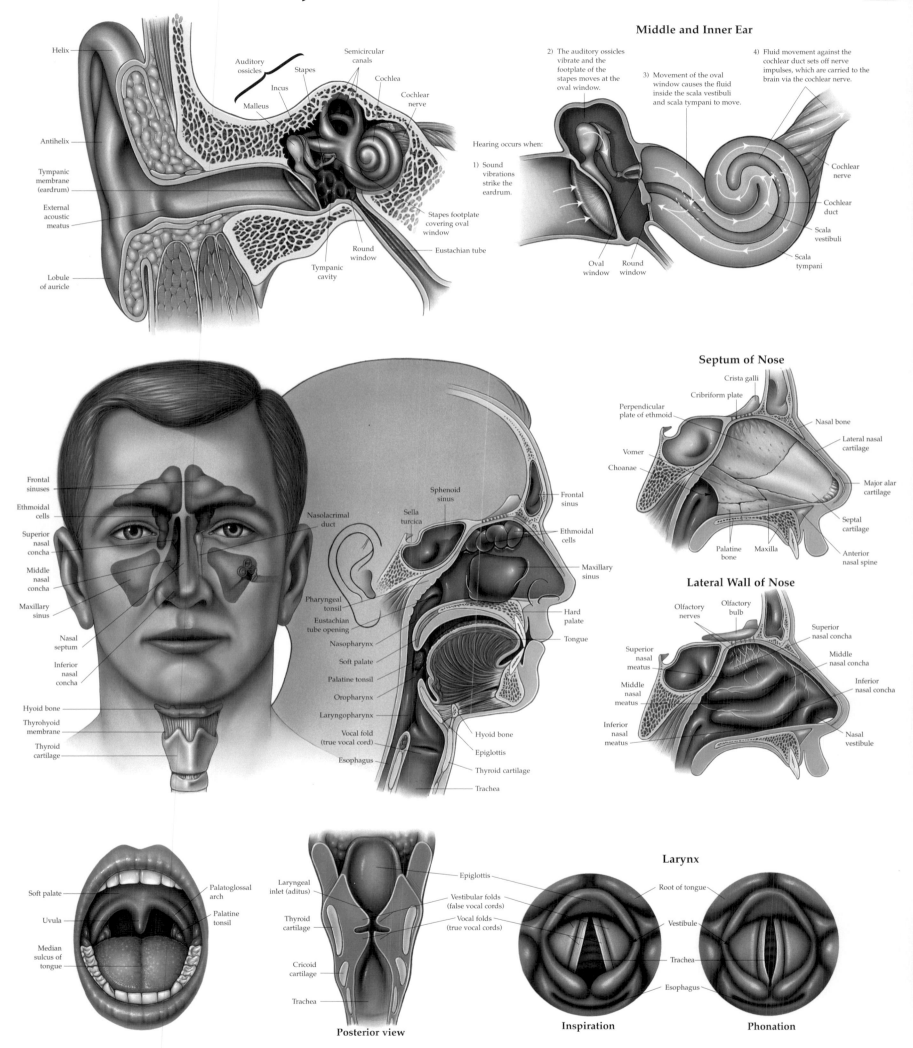

Middle and Inner Ear

Helix
Auditory ossicles
Stapes
Incus
Malleus
Semicircular canals
Cochlea
Cochlear nerve
Antihelix
Tympanic membrane (eardrum)
External acoustic meatus
Lobule of auricle
Stapes footplate covering oval window
Tympanic cavity
Round window
Eustachian tube

Hearing occurs when:

1) Sound vibrations strike the eardrum.

2) The auditory ossicles vibrate and the footplate of the stapes moves at the oval window.

3) Movement of the oval window causes the fluid inside the scala vestibuli and scala tympani to move.

4) Fluid movement against the cochlear duct sets off nerve impulses, which are carried to the brain via the cochlear nerve.

Cochlear nerve
Cochlear duct
Scala vestibuli
Scala tympani
Oval window
Round window

Septum of Nose

Crista galli
Cribriform plate
Perpendicular plate of ethmoid
Nasal bone
Lateral nasal cartilage
Vomer
Choanae
Major alar cartilage
Palatine bone
Maxilla
Septal cartilage
Anterior nasal spine

Lateral Wall of Nose

Olfactory nerves
Olfactory bulb
Superior nasal concha
Superior nasal meatus
Middle nasal concha
Middle nasal meatus
Inferior nasal concha
Inferior nasal meatus
Nasal vestibule

Frontal sinuses
Ethmoidal cells
Superior nasal concha
Middle nasal concha
Maxillary sinus
Nasal septum
Inferior nasal concha
Hyoid bone
Thyrohyoid membrane
Thyroid cartilage

Nasolacrimal duct
Sphenoid sinus
Sella turcica
Frontal sinus
Ethmoidal cells
Maxillary sinus
Pharyngeal tonsil
Eustachian tube opening
Nasopharynx
Soft palate
Palatine tonsil
Oropharynx
Laryngopharynx
Vocal fold (true vocal cord)
Esophagus
Hard palate
Tongue
Hyoid bone
Epiglottis
Thyroid cartilage
Trachea

Soft palate
Uvula
Median sulcus of tongue
Palatoglossal arch
Palatine tonsil

Larynx

Laryngeal inlet (aditus)
Thyroid cartilage
Cricoid cartilage
Trachea
Epiglottis
Vestibular folds (false vocal cords)
Vocal folds (true vocal cords)
Root of tongue
Vestibule
Trachea
Esophagus

Posterior view

Inspiration

Phonation

©2008 Wolters Kluwer | Lippincott Williams & Wilkins | Published by Anatomical Chart Company, Skokie, IL

The Eye

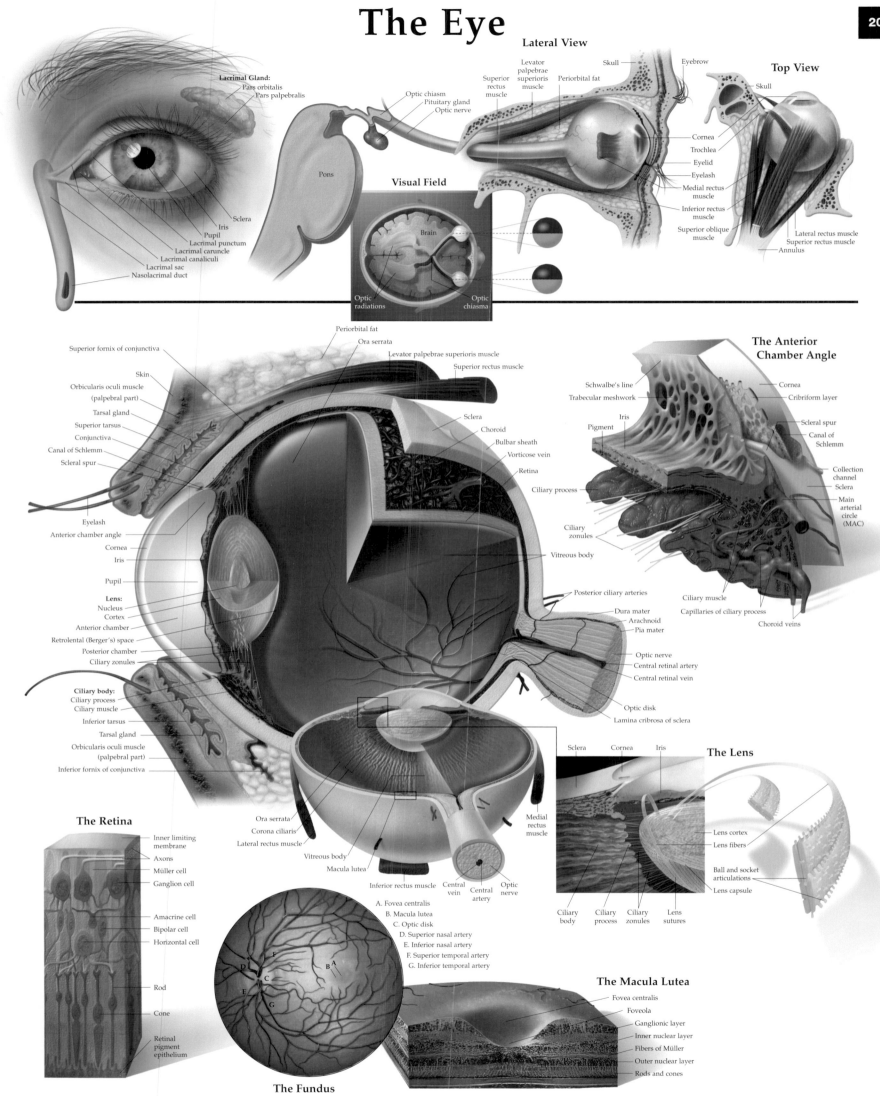

Lacrimal Gland:
Pars orbitalis
Pars palpebralis

Sclera
Iris
Pupil
Lacrimal punctum
Lacrimal caruncle
Lacrimal canaliculi
Lacrimal sac
Nasolacrimal duct

Lateral View

Levator palpebrae superioris muscle
Skull
Eyebrow
Superior rectus muscle
Periorbital fat
Optic chiasm
Pituitary gland
Optic nerve

Pons

Cornea
Trochlea
Eyelid
Eyelash
Medial rectus muscle
Inferior rectus muscle
Superior oblique muscle

Top View

Skull
Lateral rectus muscle
Superior rectus muscle
Annulus

Visual Field

Brain
Optic radiations
Optic chiasma

Periorbital fat
Ora serrata
Levator palpebrae superioris muscle
Superior rectus muscle

Superior fornix of conjunctiva
Skin
Orbicularis oculi muscle (palpebral part)
Tarsal gland
Superior tarsus
Conjunctiva
Canal of Schlemm
Scleral spur

Sclera
Choroid
Bulbar sheath
Vorticose vein
Retina

Eyelash
Anterior chamber angle
Cornea
Iris
Pupil
Lens:
Nucleus
Cortex
Anterior chamber
Retrolental (Berger's) space
Posterior chamber
Ciliary zonules

Ciliary body:
Ciliary process
Ciliary muscle
Inferior tarsus
Tarsal gland
Orbicularis oculi muscle (palpebral part)
Inferior fornix of conjunctiva

Vitreous body
Posterior ciliary arteries
Dura mater
Arachnoid
Pia mater
Optic nerve
Central retinal artery
Central retinal vein
Optic disk
Lamina cribrosa of sclera

The Anterior Chamber Angle

Schwalbe's line
Trabecular meshwork
Iris
Pigment
Ciliary process
Ciliary zonules

Cornea
Cribriform layer
Scleral spur
Canal of Schlemm
Collection channel
Sclera
Main arterial circle (MAC)
Ciliary muscle
Capillaries of ciliary process
Choroid veins

The Lens

Sclera
Cornea
Iris

Lens cortex
Lens fibers
Ball and socket articulations
Lens capsule

Ciliary body
Ciliary process
Ciliary zonules
Lens sutures

The Retina

Inner limiting membrane
Axons
Müller cell
Ganglion cell
Amacrine cell
Bipolar cell
Horizontal cell
Rod
Cone
Retinal pigment epithelium

Ora serrata
Corona ciliaris
Lateral rectus muscle
Vitreous body
Macula lutea
Inferior rectus muscle
Central vein
Central artery
Optic nerve
Medial rectus muscle

The Fundus

A. Fovea centralis
B. Macula lutea
C. Optic disk
D. Superior nasal artery
E. Inferior nasal artery
F. Superior temporal artery
G. Inferior temporal artery

The Macula Lutea

Fovea centralis
Foveola
Ganglionic layer
Inner nuclear layer
Fibers of Müller
Outer nuclear layer
Rods and cones

©2008 Wolters Kluwer Health | Lippincott Williams & Wilkins | Published by Anatomical Chart Company, Skokie, IL

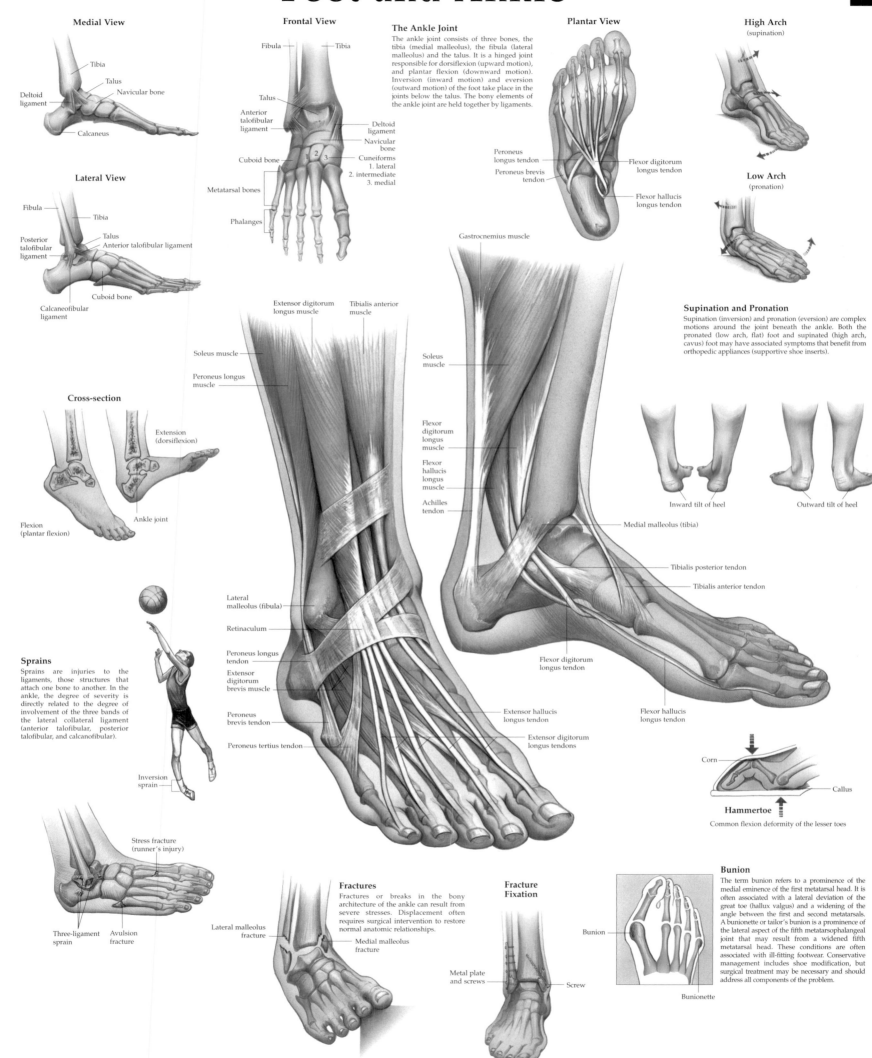

Medial View

Tibia
Talus
Navicular bone
Deltoid ligament
Calcaneus

Lateral View

Fibula
Tibia
Talus
Posterior talofibular ligament
Anterior talofibular ligament
Cuboid bone
Calcaneofibular ligament

Cross-section

Extension (dorsiflexion)
Flexion (plantar flexion)
Ankle joint

Frontal View

Fibula
Tibia
Talus
Anterior talofibular ligament
Deltoid ligament
Navicular bone
Cuboid bone
Cuneiforms
1. lateral
2. intermediate
3. medial
Metatarsal bones
Phalanges

The Ankle Joint

The ankle joint consists of three bones, the tibia (medial malleolus), the fibula (lateral malleolus) and the talus. It is a hinged joint responsible for dorsiflexion (upward motion), and plantar flexion (downward motion). Inversion (inward motion) and eversion (outward motion) of the foot take place in the joints below the talus. The bony elements of the ankle joint are held together by ligaments.

Plantar View

Peroneus longus tendon
Peroneus brevis tendon
Flexor digitorum longus tendon
Flexor hallucis longus tendon

High Arch (supination)

Low Arch (pronation)

Supination and Pronation

Supination (inversion) and pronation (eversion) are complex motions around the joint beneath the ankle. Both the pronated (low arch, flat) foot and supinated (high arch, cavus) foot may have associated symptoms that benefit from orthopedic appliances (supportive shoe inserts).

Inward tilt of heel
Outward tilt of heel

Gastrocnemius muscle
Extensor digitorum longus muscle
Tibialis anterior muscle
Soleus muscle
Peroneus longus muscle
Soleus muscle
Flexor digitorum longus muscle
Flexor hallucis longus muscle
Achilles tendon
Medial malleolus (tibia)
Tibialis posterior tendon
Tibialis anterior tendon
Lateral malleolus (fibula)
Retinaculum
Peroneus longus tendon
Extensor digitorum brevis muscle
Peroneus brevis tendon
Peroneus tertius tendon
Extensor hallucis longus tendon
Extensor digitorum longus tendons
Flexor digitorum longus tendon
Flexor hallucis longus tendon

Sprains

Sprains are injuries to the ligaments, those structures that attach one bone to another. In the ankle, the degree of severity is directly related to the degree of involvement of the three bands of the lateral collateral ligament (anterior talofibular, posterior talofibular, and calcanofibular).

Inversion sprain

Stress fracture (runner's injury)
Three-ligament sprain
Avulsion fracture

Fractures

Fractures or breaks in the bony architecture of the ankle can result from severe stresses. Displacement often requires surgical intervention to restore normal anatomic relationships.

Lateral malleolus fracture
Medial malleolus fracture

Fracture Fixation

Metal plate and screws
Screw

Corn
Callus

Hammertoe

Common flexion deformity of the lesser toes

Bunion

The term bunion refers to a prominence of the medial eminence of the first metatarsal head. It is often associated with a lateral deviation of the great toe (hallux valgus) and a widening of the angle between the first and second metatarsals. A bunionette or tailor's bunion is a prominence of the lateral aspect of the fifth metatarsophalangeal joint that may result from a widened fifth metatarsal head. These conditions are often associated with ill-fitting footwear. Conservative management includes shoe modification, but surgical treatment may be necessary and should address all components of the problem.

Bunion
Bunionette

©2008 Wolters Kluwer Health | Lippincott Williams & Wilkins | Published by Anatomical Chart Company, Skokie, IL

Hand and Wrist

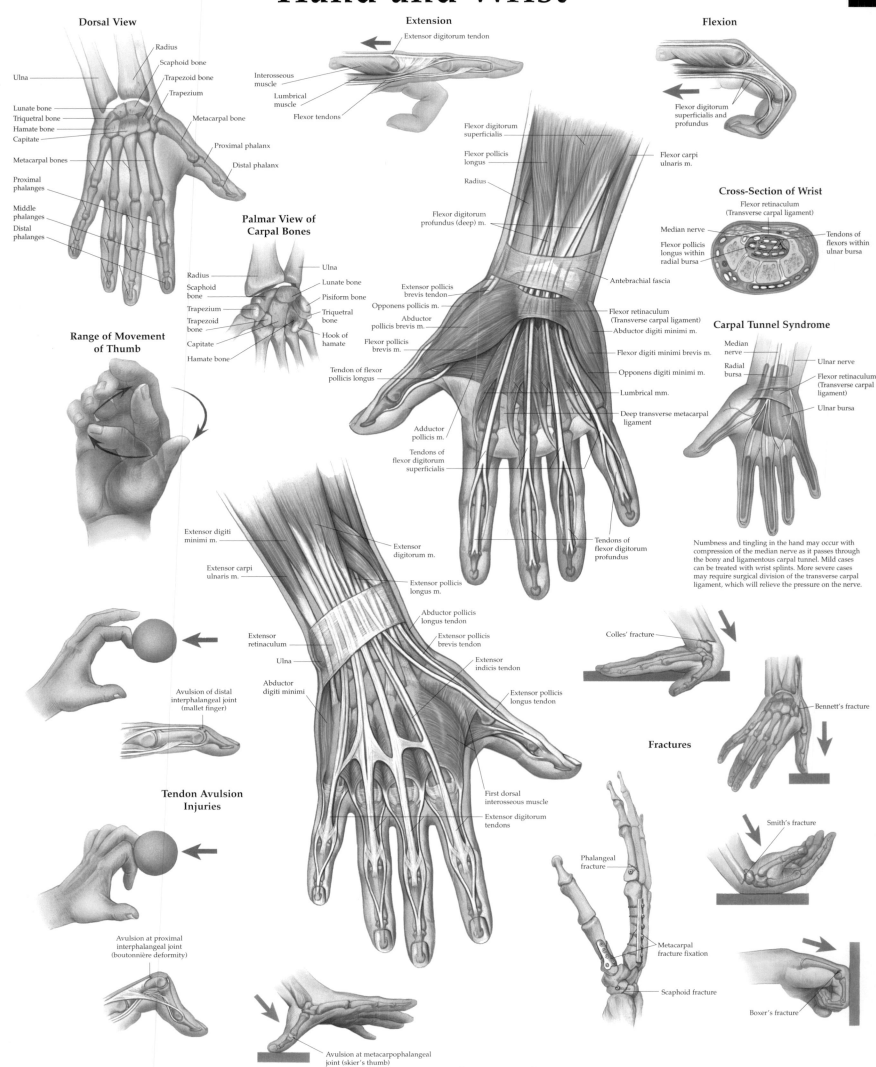

Dorsal View

- Radius
- Scaphoid bone
- Trapezoid bone
- Trapezium
- Ulna
- Lunate bone
- Triquetral bone
- Hamate bone
- Capitate
- Metacarpal bone
- Metacarpal bones
- Proximal phalanx
- Distal phalanx
- Proximal phalanges
- Middle phalanges
- Distal phalanges

Extension

- Extensor digitorum tendon
- Interosseous muscle
- Lumbrical muscle
- Flexor tendons

Flexion

- Flexor digitorum superficialis and profundus

Palmar View of Carpal Bones

- Radius
- Ulna
- Scaphoid bone
- Lunate bone
- Pisiform bone
- Trapezium
- Triquetral bone
- Trapezoid bone
- Hook of hamate
- Capitate
- Hamate bone

Range of Movement of Thumb

- Flexor digitorum superficialis
- Flexor pollicis longus
- Radius
- Flexor digitorum profundus (deep) m.
- Extensor pollicis brevis tendon
- Opponens pollicis m.
- Abductor pollicis brevis m.
- Flexor pollicis brevis m.
- Tendon of flexor pollicis longus
- Adductor pollicis m.
- Tendons of flexor digitorum superficialis
- Flexor carpi ulnaris m.
- Antebrachial fascia
- Flexor retinaculum (Transverse carpal ligament)
- Abductor digiti minimi m.
- Flexor digiti minimi brevis m.
- Opponens digiti minimi m.
- Lumbrical mm.
- Deep transverse metacarpal ligament
- Tendons of flexor digitorum profundus

Cross-Section of Wrist

- Flexor retinaculum (Transverse carpal ligament)
- Median nerve
- Flexor pollicis longus within radial bursa
- Tendons of flexors within ulnar bursa

Carpal Tunnel Syndrome

- Median nerve
- Radial bursa
- Ulnar nerve
- Flexor retinaculum (Transverse carpal ligament)
- Ulnar bursa

Numbness and tingling in the hand may occur with compression of the median nerve as it passes through the bony and ligamentous carpal tunnel. Mild cases can be treated with wrist splints. More severe cases may require surgical division of the transverse carpal ligament, which will relieve the pressure on the nerve.

- Extensor digiti minimi m.
- Extensor digitorum m.
- Extensor carpi ulnaris m.
- Extensor pollicis longus m.
- Extensor retinaculum
- Abductor pollicis longus tendon
- Extensor pollicis brevis tendon
- Ulna
- Extensor indicis tendon
- Abductor digiti minimi
- Extensor pollicis longus tendon
- First dorsal interosseous muscle
- Extensor digitorum tendons

Tendon Avulsion Injuries

- Avulsion of distal interphalangeal joint (mallet finger)
- Avulsion at proximal interphalangeal joint (boutonnière deformity)
- Avulsion at metacarpophalangeal joint (skier's thumb)

Fractures

- Colles' fracture
- Bennett's fracture
- Smith's fracture
- Phalangeal fracture
- Metacarpal fracture fixation
- Scaphoid fracture
- Boxer's fracture

©2008 Wolters Kluwer Health | Lippincott Williams & Wilkins | Published by Anatomical Chart Company, Skokie, IL

The Heart

Thorax

- Manubrium
- 2nd rib
- Sternum
- Heart
- 5th rib
- Diaphragm
- Xiphoid process

1. Right brachiocephalic v.
2. Left brachiocephalic v.
3. Brachiocephalic trunk
4. Left common carotid a.
5. Left subclavian a.
6. Superior vena cava
7. Arch of aorta
8. Ligamentum arteriosum
9. Pulmonary trunk
10. Right atrium
11. Right auricle
12. Pulmonary valve
    a) anterior semilunar cusp
    b) right semilunar cusp
    c) left semilunar cusp
13. Right coronary a.
14. Right ventricle (opened)
15. Right atrioventricular (A-V valve) (tricuspid)
16. Chordae tendineae
17. Papillary muscles
18. Trabeculae
19. Muscular wall of right ventricle
20. Right marginal a.
21. Small cardiac v.
22. Pericardial sac
23. Auricle of left atrium
24. Left coronary a.
25. Circumflex a.
26. Left marginal a.
27. Diagonal a.
28. Anterior interventricular a.
29. Great cardiac v.
30. Left ventricle
31. Apex of heart
32. Diaphragm

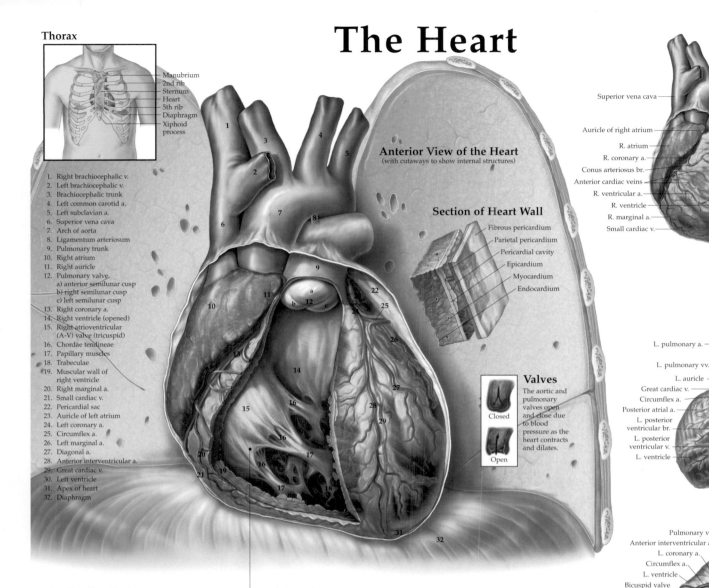

Anterior View of the Heart
(with cutaways to show internal structures)

Section of Heart Wall

- Fibrous pericardium
- Parietal pericardium
- Pericardial cavity
- Epicardium
- Myocardium
- Endocardium

Valves

The aortic and pulmonary valves open and close due to blood pressure as the heart contracts and dilates.

Closed

Open

Anterior View

- Superior vena cava
- Auricle of right atrium
- R. atrium
- R. coronary a.
- Conus arteriosus br.
- Anterior cardiac veins
- R. ventricular a.
- R. ventricle
- R. marginal a.
- Small cardiac v.
- L. pulmonary a.
- Aorta
- Pulmonary trunk
- Auricle of left atrium
- L. coronary a.
- L. marginal a.
- Diagonal a.
- Anterior interventricular a.
- Great cardiac v.
- L. ventricle
- Apex

Posterior View

- Superior vena cava
- Aortic arch
- L. pulmonary a.
- L. pulmonary vv.
- L. auricle
- Great cardiac v.
- Circumflex a.
- Posterior atrial a.
- L. posterior ventricular br.
- L. posterior ventricular v.
- L. ventricle
- R. pulmonary a.
- L. atrium
- R. pulmonary vv.
- R. atrium
- Oblique vv.
- Inferior vena cava
- Small cardiac v.
- R. coronary a.
- Coronary sinus
- R. posterior interventricular aa.
- Middle cardiac v.
- R. ventricle

Heart Valves

(anterior)

- Pulmonary valve
- Anterior interventricular a.
- L. coronary a.
- Circumflex a.
- L. ventricle
- Bicuspid valve (mitral valve)
- Great cardiac v.
- Coronary sinus
- Aortic valve
- R. coronary a.
- Conus arteriosus br.
- R. marginal a.
- Tricuspid valve

(posterior)

Key
- a. anterior
- b. posterior
- c. left
- d. right
- e. septal

The Cardiac Cycle

Heart muscles contract (systole) and dilate (diastole) in a repeating cardiac cycle. The cycle or "heartbeat" occurs approximately 70 times per minute, pumping blood through the heart and to the body. During this cycle, deoxygenated blood enters the right side of the heart from the body and is pumped into the lungs. Oxygenated blood from the lungs enters the left side of the heart and is pumped out to the body. The illustration below demonstrates this sequence of events.

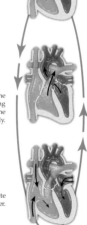

①

Atrial Systole

The atria contract, emptying blood into the ventricles.

②

Ventricular Systole

Shortly after atrial systole, the ventricles contract, ejecting blood from the heart to the lungs and the rest of the body.

③

Diastole

Atria and ventricles dilate and blood refills each chamber.

Key: Abbreviations

Artery – a.
Arteries – aa.
Vein – v.
Veins – vv.
Branch – br.
Right – R.
Left – L.

A-V Valves

As the heart contracts, the A-V valves (mitral and tricuspid) close. Chordae tendineae and papillary muscles work together to keep the valve from prolapsing into the atrium.

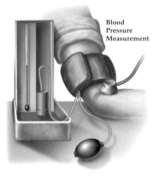

Open

Closed

Blood Pressure Measurement

Blood Pressure (BP)

As blood is pumped through the body, it creates pressure within the arteries. This pressure is referred to as blood pressure. A blood pressure reading indicates arterial pressure during the heart's contraction (systole) and dilation (diastole). Blood pressure measurement is an important tool to assess the functioning of the heart, kidneys, and blood vessels.

Normal BP

$$\frac{\text{Systolic mmHg}}{\text{Diastolic mmHg}} < \frac{130 \text{ mmHg}}{85 \text{ mmHg}}$$

Low BP

$$\frac{\text{Systolic mmHg}}{\text{Diastolic mmHg}} < \frac{80 \text{ mmHg}}{60 \text{ mmHg}}$$

High BP

$$\frac{\text{Systolic mmHg}}{\text{Diastolic mmHg}} > \frac{140 \text{ mmHg}}{90 \text{ mmHg}}$$

Coronary Arteries
(anterior view)

Coronary arteries supply blood to heart tissue. They originate from the aorta.

- Aorta
- Br. to S-A node
- R. coronary a.
- R. atrial aa.
- Conus arteriosus br.
- R. anterior ventricular a.
- R. marginal a.
- R. posterior interventricular a.
- L. coronary a.
- Circumflex a.
- Posterior atrial a.
- L. marginal a.
- Diagonal a.
- Anterior interventricular a.
- L. posterior ventricular br.

● *Common areas of coronary artery blockage that result in damage to heart muscle.*

Cardiac Conduction

Repeating electrical impulses travel through the heart, controlling the rhythmic contraction and dilation of the heart muscle.

A. The impulse originates from the Sinoatrial (S-A) node, located in the right atrium, and spreads across the atria, causing them to contract.

B. The impulse then passes to the atrioventricular (A-V) node, travels along the atrioventricular bundle, into the right and left crura and spreads into the ventricles, causing them to contract.

C. As the impulse dissipates, the atria and ventricles relax (dilate).

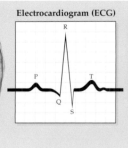

Sinoatrial (S-A) node 1.
Interatrial septum 2.
Atrioventricular (A-V) node 3.
Atrioventricular bundle 4. (bundle of His)
Right crus 5.
Left crus 6.
Interventricular septum 7.
Purkinje's fibers 8.

Electrocardiogram (ECG)

An electrocardiogram (ECG) is a record of the electrical activity of the heart as the impulse travels from the atria through the ventricles. This record is displayed in a waveform with three distinct waves: P, QRS and T.

Hip and Knee

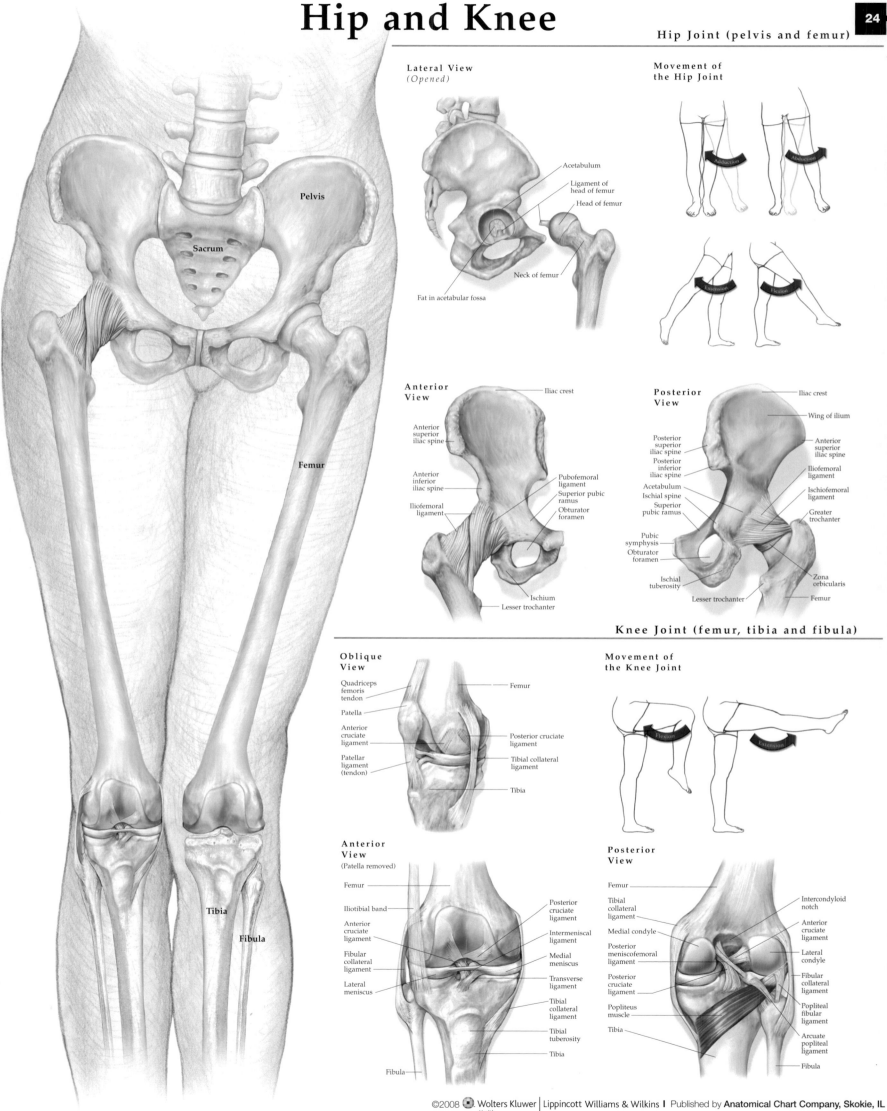

Lateral View *(Opened)*

- Acetabulum
- Ligament of head of femur
- Head of femur
- Neck of femur
- Fat in acetabular fossa

Movement of the Hip Joint

Adduction · Abduction

Extension · Flexion

Anterior View

- Iliac crest
- Anterior superior iliac spine
- Anterior inferior iliac spine
- Iliofemoral ligament
- Pubofemoral ligament
- Superior pubic ramus
- Obturator foramen
- Ischium
- Lesser trochanter

Posterior View

- Iliac crest
- Wing of ilium
- Posterior superior iliac spine
- Posterior inferior iliac spine
- Anterior superior iliac spine
- Acetabulum
- Iliofemoral ligament
- Ischial spine
- Ischiofemoral ligament
- Superior pubic ramus
- Greater trochanter
- Pubic symphysis
- Obturator foramen
- Ischial tuberosity
- Zona orbicularis
- Lesser trochanter
- Femur

Knee Joint (femur, tibia and fibula)

Oblique View

- Quadriceps femoris tendon
- Patella
- Anterior cruciate ligament
- Patellar ligament (tendon)
- Femur
- Posterior cruciate ligament
- Tibial collateral ligament
- Tibia

Movement of the Knee Joint

Flexion · Extension

Anterior View (Patella removed)

- Femur
- Iliotibial band
- Anterior cruciate ligament
- Fibular collateral ligament
- Lateral meniscus
- Posterior cruciate ligament
- Intermeniscal ligament
- Medial meniscus
- Transverse ligament
- Tibial collateral ligament
- Tibial tuberosity
- Tibia
- Fibula

Posterior View

- Femur
- Tibial collateral ligament
- Medial condyle
- Posterior meniscofemoral ligament
- Posterior cruciate ligament
- Popliteus muscle
- Tibia
- Intercondyloid notch
- Anterior cruciate ligament
- Lateral condyle
- Fibular collateral ligament
- Popliteal fibular ligament
- Arcuate popliteal ligament
- Fibula

Pelvis · Sacrum · Femur · Tibia · Fibula

©2008 Wolters Kluwer | Lippincott Williams & Wilkins | Published by Anatomical Chart Company, Skokie, IL

Internal Organs of the Human Body

The brain is the command center of the central nervous system. It receives signals that tell the body what to do and controls both voluntary and involuntary activities. The brain is the home of emotion, memory, thought, and language.

The lungs are the main component of the respiratory system. They distribute air and exchange gases, removing carbon dioxide from the blood and providing it with oxygen.

The heart pumps the body's entire volume of blood to and from the lungs (using the right ventricle and left atrium) and to and from all the organs (using the left ventricle and right atrium).

The diaphragm plays a vital role in breathing. As it contracts and flattens, it helps draw air into the lungs; as it relaxes, it helps push the air out of the lungs.

The liver, the largest internal organ performs complex and important functions related to digestion and nutrition. The liver produces bile (which helps break down food matter in the small intestine), detoxifies blood, helps regulate blood glucose levels, and produces plasma proteins.

The kidneys eliminate waste, filter blood, maintain fluid-electrolyte and acid-base balances, produce the hormone that stimulates the production of red blood cells, produce enzymes that govern blood pressure, and help activate vitamin D.

The spleen breaks down old red blood cells and selectively retains and destroys damaged or abnormal red blood cells. It also filters out bacteria and other foreign substances that enter the bloodstream. The spleen stores blood and produces cells involved in immune response.

The gallbladder stores the bile that is secreted by the liver.

The pancreas assists with the digestion of many substances such as protein, nucleic acids, starch, fats and cholesterol. Using the hormone insulin, the pancreas controls the amount of sugar stored in and released from the liver for use throughout the body.

The stomach temporarily stores food and begins the digestion process, breaking down the food with gastric acids and moving it into the small intestine.

The large intestine absorbs water, secretes mucus, and eliminates digestive waste.

The small intestine completes digestion. Food molecules are absorbed through the wall of the intestine into the circulatory system and delivered to the cells of the body.

The bladder stores urine that has been excreted from the kidney.

Brain

Lung

Lung

Heart

Liver

Diaphragm

Kidney *(outlined)*

Gallbladder *(outlined)*

Pancreas

Stomach

Kidney *(outlined)*

Spleen

Large intestine (Colon)

Small intestine

Bladder

©2008 Wolters Kluwer Health | Lippincott Williams & Wilkins | Published by Anatomical Chart Company, Skokie, IL

Ligaments of the Joints

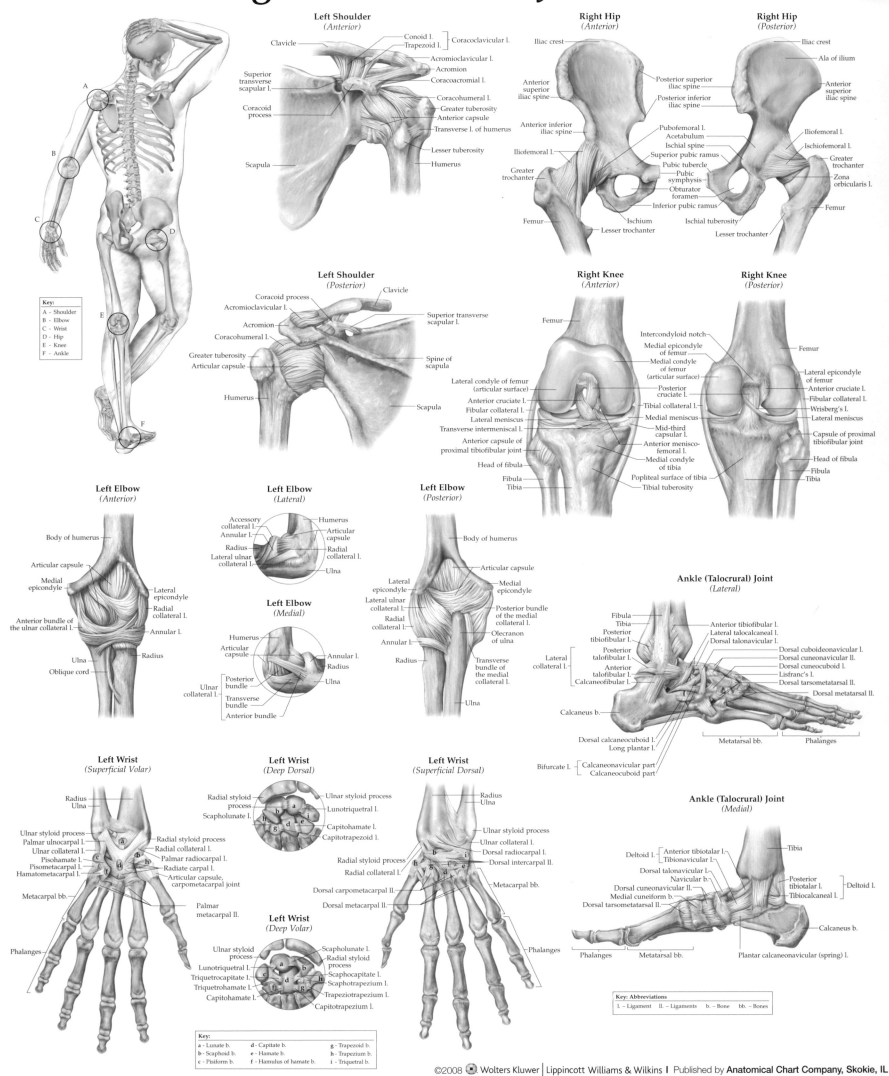

Key:
A - Shoulder
B - Elbow
C - Wrist
D - Hip
E - Knee
F - Ankle

Left Shoulder
(Anterior)

Clavicle · Conoid l. Trapezoid l.] Coracoclavicular l. · Acromioclavicular l. · Acromion · Coracoacromial l. · Coracohumeral l. · Greater tuberosity · Anterior capsule · Transverse l. of humerus · Lesser tuberosity · Humerus · Superior transverse scapular l. · Coracoid process · Scapula

Right Hip
(Anterior)

Iliac crest · Anterior superior iliac spine · Anterior inferior iliac spine · Iliofemoral l. · Greater trochanter · Femur · Posterior superior iliac spine · Posterior inferior iliac spine · Pubofemoral l. · Acetabulum · Ischial spine · Superior pubic ramus · Pubic tubercle · Pubic symphysis · Obturator foramen · Inferior pubic ramus · Ischium · Lesser trochanter · Ischial tuberosity

Right Hip
(Posterior)

Iliac crest · Ala of ilium · Anterior superior iliac spine · Iliofemoral l. · Ischiofemoral l. · Greater trochanter · Zona orbicularis l. · Femur · Lesser trochanter

Left Shoulder
(Posterior)

Coracoid process · Acromioclavicular l. · Acromion · Coracohumeral l. · Greater tuberosity · Articular capsule · Humerus · Clavicle · Superior transverse scapular l. · Spine of scapula · Scapula

Right Knee
(Anterior)

Femur · Lateral condyle of femur (articular surface) · Anterior cruciate l. · Fibular collateral l. · Lateral meniscus · Transverse intermeniscal l. · Anterior capsule of proximal tibiofibular joint · Head of fibula · Fibula · Tibia · Intercondyloid notch · Medial epicondyle of femur · Medial condyle of femur (articular surface) · Posterior cruciate · Tibial collateral l. · Medial meniscus · Mid-third capsular l. · Anterior menisco-femoral l. · Medial condyle of tibia · Popliteal surface of tibia · Tibial tuberosity

Right Knee
(Posterior)

Femur · Lateral epicondyle of femur · Anterior cruciate l. · Fibular collateral l. · Wrisberg's l. · Lateral meniscus · Capsule of proximal tibiofibular joint · Head of fibula · Fibula · Tibia

Left Elbow
(Anterior)

Body of humerus · Articular capsule · Medial epicondyle · Anterior bundle of the ulnar collateral l. · Ulna · Oblique cord · Lateral epicondyle · Radial collateral l. · Annular l. · Radius

Left Elbow
(Lateral)

Accessory collateral l. · Annular l. · Radius · Lateral ulnar collateral l. · Humerus · Articular capsule · Radial collateral l. · Ulna

Left Elbow
(Medial)

Humerus · Articular capsule · Ulnar collateral l. · Posterior bundle · Transverse bundle · Anterior bundle · Annular l. · Radius · Ulna

Left Elbow
(Posterior)

Lateral epicondyle · Lateral ulnar collateral l. · Radial collateral l. · Annular l. · Radius · Body of humerus · Articular capsule · Medial epicondyle · Posterior bundle of the medial collateral l. · Olecranon of ulna · Transverse bundle of the medial collateral l. · Ulna

Ankle (Talocrural) Joint
(Lateral)

Fibula · Tibia · Posterior tibiofibular l. · Posterior talofibular l. · Anterior talofibular l. · Calcaneofibular l. · Calcaneus b. · Dorsal calcaneocuboid l. · Long plantar l. · Bifurcate l. · Calcaneonavicular part · Calcaneocuboid part · Anterior tibiofibular l. · Lateral talocalcaneal l. · Dorsal talonavicular l. · Dorsal cuboideonavicular l. · Dorsal cuneonavicular ll. · Dorsal cuneocuboid l. · Lisfranc's l. · Dorsal tarsometatarsal ll. · Dorsal metatarsal l. · Lateral collateral l. · Metatarsal bb. · Phalanges

Left Wrist
(Superficial Volar)

Radius · Ulna · Ulnar styloid process · Palmar ulnocarpal l. · Ulnar collateral l. · Pisohamate l. · Pisometacarpal l. · Hamatometacarpal l. · Metacarpal bb. · Phalanges · Radial styloid process · Radial collateral l. · Palmar radiocarpal l. · Radiate carpal l. · Articular capsule, carpometacarpal joint · Palmar metacarpal ll.

Left Wrist
(Deep Dorsal)

Radial styloid process · Scapholunate l. · Ulnar styloid process · Lunotriquetral l. · Capitohamate l. · Capitotrapezoid l.

Left Wrist
(Superficial Dorsal)

Radial styloid process · Radial collateral l. · Dorsal carpometacarpal ll. · Dorsal metacarpal ll. · Radius · Ulna · Ulnar styloid process · Ulnar collateral l. · Dorsal radiocarpal l. · Dorsal intercarpal ll. · Metacarpal bb. · Phalanges

Left Wrist
(Deep Volar)

Ulnar styloid process · Lunotriquetral l. · Triquetrocapitate l. · Triquetrohamate l. · Capitohamate l. · Scapholunate l. · Radial styloid process · Scaphocapitate l. · Scaphotrapezium l. · Trapeziotrapezium l. · Capitotrapezium l.

Ankle (Talocrural) Joint
(Medial)

Deltoid l. · Anterior tibiotalar l. · Dorsal talonavicular l. · Navicular b. · Dorsal cuneonavicular ll. · Medial cuneiform b. · Dorsal tarsometatarsal ll. · Phalanges · Metatarsal bb. · Tibia · Posterior tibiotalar l. · Tibiocalcaneal l.] Deltoid l. · Calcaneus b. · Plantar calcaneonavicular (spring) l.

Key: Abbreviations
l. – Ligament   ll. – Ligaments   b. – Bone   bb. – Bones

Key:
a - Lunate b.   d - Capitate b.   g - Trapezoid b.
b - Scaphoid b.   e - Hamate b.   h - Trapezium b.
c - Pisiform b.   f - Hamulus of hamate b.   i - Triquetral b.

©2008 Wolters Kluwer Health | Lippincott Williams & Wilkins | Published by Anatomical Chart Company, Skokie, IL

Pregnancy and Birth

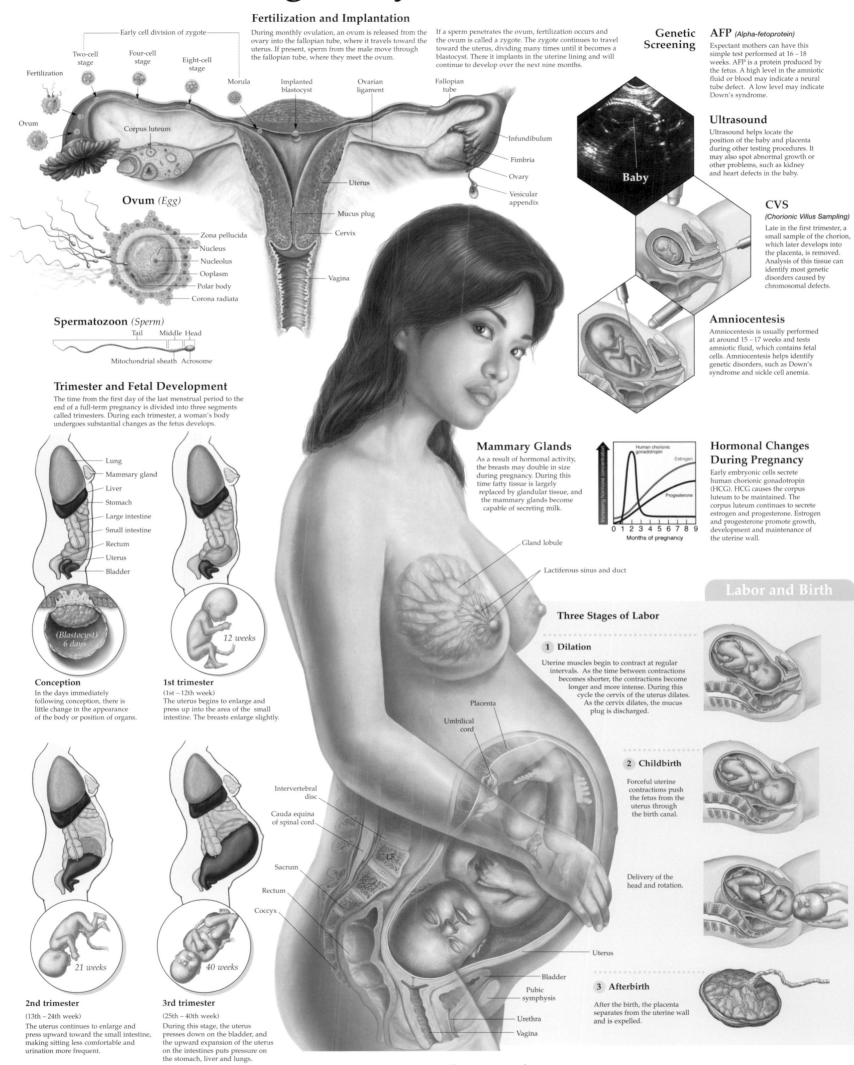

Fertilization and Implantation

During monthly ovulation, an ovum is released from the ovary into the fallopian tube, where it travels toward the uterus. If present, sperm from the male move through the fallopian tube, where they meet the ovum.

If a sperm penetrates the ovum, fertilization occurs and the ovum is called a zygote. The zygote continues to travel toward the uterus, dividing many times until it becomes a blastocyst. There it implants in the uterine lining and will continue to develop over the next nine months.

Early cell division of zygote
Two-cell stage
Four-cell stage
Eight-cell stage
Fertilization
Morula
Ovum
Implanted blastocyst
Ovarian ligament
Fallopian tube
Corpus luteum
Infundibulum
Fimbria
Ovary
Vesicular appendix
Uterus
Mucus plug
Cervix
Vagina

Ovum (Egg)

Zona pellucida
Nucleus
Nucleolus
Ooplasm
Polar body
Corona radiata

Spermatozoon (Sperm)

Tail
Middle
Head
Mitochondrial sheath
Acrosome

Trimester and Fetal Development

The time from the first day of the last menstrual period to the end of a full-term pregnancy is divided into three segments called trimesters. During each trimester, a woman's body undergoes substantial changes as the fetus develops.

Lung
Mammary gland
Liver
Stomach
Large intestine
Small intestine
Rectum
Uterus
Bladder

(Blastocyst) 6 days

12 weeks

Conception
In the days immediately following conception, there is little change in the appearance of the body or position of organs.

1st trimester
(1st – 12th week)
The uterus begins to enlarge and press up into the area of the small intestine. The breasts enlarge slightly.

21 weeks

40 weeks

Intervertebral disc
Cauda equina of spinal cord
L3
Sacrum
Rectum
Coccyx

2nd trimester
(13th – 24th week)
The uterus continues to enlarge and press upward toward the small intestine, making sitting less comfortable and urination more frequent.

3rd trimester
(25th – 40th week)
During this stage, the uterus presses down on the bladder, and the upward expansion of the uterus on the intestines puts pressure on the stomach, liver and lungs.

Genetic Screening

AFP (Alpha-fetoprotein)
Expectant mothers can have this simple test performed at 16 – 18 weeks. AFP is a protein produced by the fetus. A high level in the amniotic fluid or blood may indicate a neural tube defect. A low level may indicate Down's syndrome.

Ultrasound
Ultrasound helps locate the position of the baby and placenta during other testing procedures. It may also spot abnormal growth or other problems, such as kidney and heart defects in the baby.

Baby

CVS
(Chorionic Villus Sampling)
Late in the first trimester, a small sample of the chorion, which later develops into the placenta, is removed. Analysis of this tissue can identify most genetic disorders caused by chromosomal defects.

Amniocentesis
Amniocentesis is usually performed at around 15 – 17 weeks and tests amniotic fluid, which contains fetal cells. Amniocentesis helps identify genetic disorders, such as Down's syndrome and sickle cell anemia.

Mammary Glands
As a result of hormonal activity, the breasts may double in size during pregnancy. During this time fatty tissue is largely replaced by glandular tissue, and the mammary glands become capable of secreting milk.

Gland lobule
Lactiferous sinus and duct

Hormonal Changes During Pregnancy
Early embryonic cells secrete human chorionic gonadotropin (HCG). HCG causes the corpus luteum to be maintained. The corpus luteum continues to secrete estrogen and progesterone. Estrogen and progesterone promote growth, development and maintenance of the uterine wall.

Human chorionic gonadotropin
Estrogen
Progesterone
Increasing hormone concentration
0 1 2 3 4 5 6 7 8 9
Months of pregnancy

Placenta
Umbilical cord
Bladder
Pubic symphysis
Urethra
Vagina
Uterus

Labor and Birth

Three Stages of Labor

1 Dilation
Uterine muscles begin to contract at regular intervals. As the time between contractions becomes shorter, the contractions become longer and more intense. During this cycle the cervix of the uterus dilates. As the cervix dilates, the mucus plug is discharged.

2 Childbirth
Forceful uterine contractions push the fetus from the uterus through the birth canal.

Delivery of the head and rotation.

3 Afterbirth
After the birth, the placenta separates from the uterine wall and is expelled.

©2008 Wolters Kluwer Health | Lippincott Williams & Wilkins | Published by Anatomical Chart Company, Skokie, IL

The Prostate

Hormonal Influence on the Prostate

The prostate functions continuously, producing fluid which empties into the urethra. Hormones from the **pituitary gland** direct the **adrenal glands** and the **testes** to send chemical signals to the **prostate** to promote fluid production.

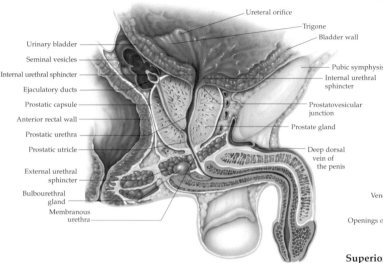

- Pituitary
- Adrenal gland
- Kidney
- Ureter
- Urinary bladder
- Prostate
- Testis

What is the Prostate?

The prostate is a gland consisting of fibrous, muscular and glandular tissue surrounding the urethra below the urinary bladder. Its function is to secrete prostatic fluid as a medium for semen, helping it to reach the female reproductive tract. Within the prostate, the urethra is joined by two ejaculatory ducts. During sexual activity, the prostate acts as a valve between the urinary and reproductive tracts. This enables semen to ejaculate without mixing with urine. Prostatic fluid is delivered by the contraction of muscles around gland tissue. Nerve and hormonal influences control the secretory and muscular functions of the prostate.

Normal Prostate (sagittal section)

Labels:
- Ureteral orifice
- Trigone
- Bladder wall
- Urinary bladder
- Seminal vesicles
- Internal urethral sphincter
- Ejaculatory ducts
- Prostatic capsule
- Anterior rectal wall
- Prostatic urethra
- Prostatic utricle
- External urethral sphincter
- Bulbourethral gland
- Membranous urethra
- Pubic symphysis
- Internal urethral sphincter
- Prostatovesicular junction
- Prostate gland
- Deep dorsal vein of the penis

Posterior View (dissected)

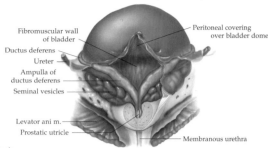

- Fibromuscular wall of bladder
- Ductus deferens
- Ureter
- Ampulla of ductus deferens
- Seminal vesicles
- Levator ani m.
- Prostatic utricle
- Peritoneal covering over bladder dome
- Membranous urethra

Anterior View with Exposed Prostatic Urethra

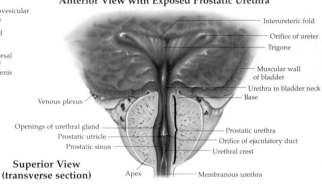

- Interureteric fold
- Orifice of ureter
- Trigone
- Muscular wall of bladder
- Urethra in bladder neck
- Base
- Venous plexus
- Openings of urethral gland
- Prostatic utricle
- Prostatic sinus
- Apex
- Prostatic urethra
- Orifice of ejaculatory duct
- Urethral crest
- Membranous urethra

Superior View (transverse section)

- Prostate glandular tissue lobes
- Prostatic urethra
- Prostatic utricle
- Ejaculatory ducts

Vasculature and Innervation

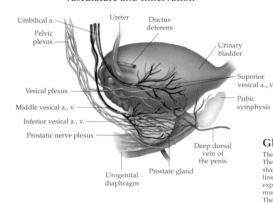

- Umbilical a.
- Pelvic plexus
- Ureter
- Ductus deferens
- Urinary bladder
- Vesical plexus
- Superior vesical a., v.
- Middle vesical a., v.
- Inferior vesical a., v.
- Prostatic nerve plexus
- Pubic symphysis
- Urogenital diaphragm
- Prostate gland
- Deep dorsal vein of the penis

Zones of the Prostate

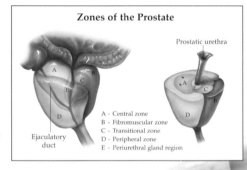

- Prostatic urethra
- Ejaculatory duct

A - Central zone
B - Fibromuscular zone
C - Transitional zone
D - Peripheral zone
E - Periurethral gland region

Glands of the Prostate

The prostate is mainly filled with secretory glands. These glands are made of many ducts with grape-shaped saccule ends or "acini". Secretory cells lining the ducts are stimulated by hormones to expel prostatic fluid. During sexual activity muscle contracts and secrete prostatic fluid. The basal cell, also found lining the ducts of the prostate, may be responsible for most types of prostatic hyperplasia as a result of uncontrolled prostatic tissue growth.

Secretory gland with grape-shaped **acinus** end.

- Prostatic duct
- **Secretory cells** are the most numerous in the gland and form the inner lining.
- The **basal cell** is located below the lining surface and may function to rebuild prostatic tissue after infection or other damage.
- Fibromuscular stroma
- Ductal lumen
- Prostatic fluid

Benign Prostatic Hyperplasia (BPH)

Benign Prostatic Hyperplasia (BPH), is the most common type of tumor in mature men. It is a benign growth, which means it may enlarge but will not spread to other locations in the body. The tumor can cause discomfort and may grow to completely close the bladder neck, preventing urination. This condition occurs because the tumor usually grows in the transitional zone and periurethral gland region located at the prostate base near the bladder neck.

Early BPH:

Narrowing of the prostatic urethra causing difficulty in starting, maintaining, and stopping urination.

- Prostatic urethra

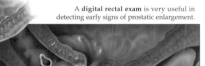

Prostatitis

Prostatitis is an uncomfortable condition in which the prostate becomes inflamed and swollen due to an infection. Prostatitis can make urinating painful.

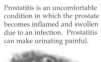
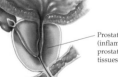

- Prostatis (inflamed prostate tissues)

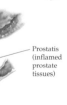

A **digital rectal exam** is very useful in detecting early signs of prostatic enlargement.

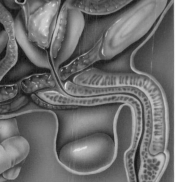

Prostate Cancer

Prostate carcinoma is the most common malignant tumor in men. Unlike BPH, prostate cancer not only enlarges but also metastasizes (spreads) to other parts of the body through lymphatic and venous channels.

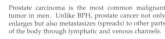
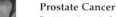
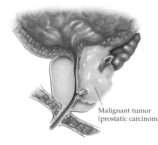

- Malignant tumor (prostatic carcinoma)

Pathways of Prostate Cancer Spread

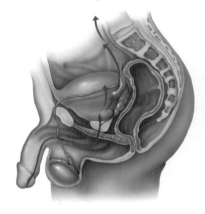

Shoulder and Elbow

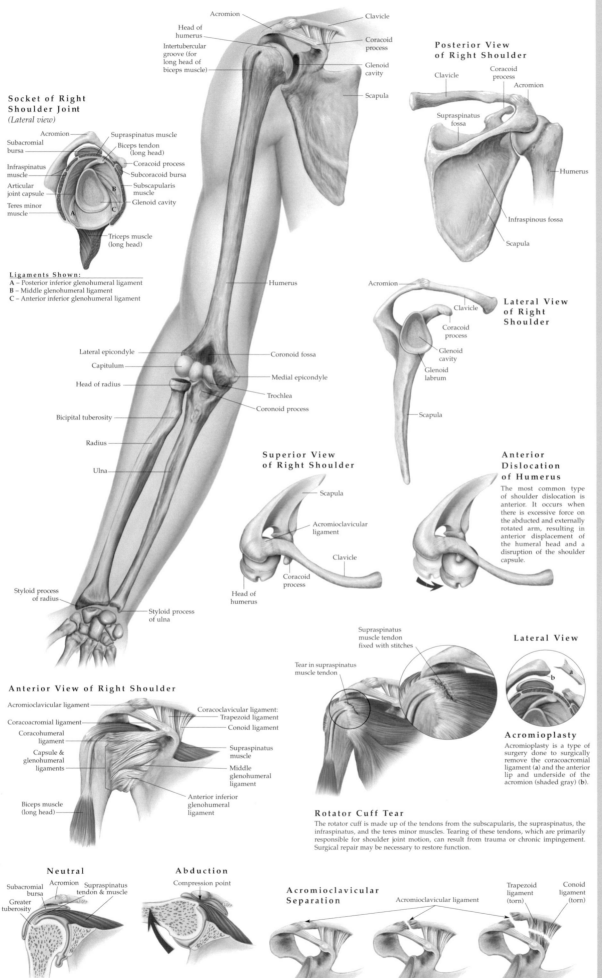

Socket of Right Shoulder Joint *(Lateral view)*

- Acromion
- Subacromial bursa
- Infraspinatus muscle
- Articular joint capsule
- Teres minor muscle
- Supraspinatus muscle
- Biceps tendon (long head)
- Coracoid process
- Subcoracoid bursa
- Subscapularis muscle
- Glenoid cavity
- Triceps muscle (long head)

Ligaments Shown:
A – Posterior inferior glenohumeral ligament
B – Middle glenohumeral ligament
C – Anterior inferior glenohumeral ligament

Labels on central arm figure:
- Acromion
- Head of humerus
- Intertubercular groove (for long head of biceps muscle)
- Clavicle
- Coracoid process
- Glenoid cavity
- Scapula
- Humerus
- Lateral epicondyle
- Capitulum
- Head of radius
- Bicipital tuberosity
- Radius
- Ulna
- Coronoid fossa
- Medial epicondyle
- Trochlea
- Coronoid process
- Styloid process of radius
- Styloid process of ulna

Posterior View of Right Shoulder
- Clavicle
- Coracoid process
- Acromion
- Supraspinatus fossa
- Humerus
- Infraspinous fossa
- Scapula

Lateral View of Right Shoulder
- Acromion
- Clavicle
- Coracoid process
- Glenoid cavity
- Glenoid labrum
- Scapula

Superior View of Right Shoulder
- Scapula
- Acromioclavicular ligament
- Clavicle
- Coracoid process
- Head of humerus

Anterior Dislocation of Humerus

The most common type of shoulder dislocation is anterior. It occurs when there is excessive force on the abducted and externally rotated arm, resulting in anterior displacement of the humeral head and a disruption of the shoulder capsule.

Anterior View of Right Shoulder
- Acromioclavicular ligament
- Coracoacromial ligament
- Coracohumeral ligament
- Capsule & glenohumeral ligaments
- Biceps muscle (long head)
- Coracoclavicular ligament: Trapezoid ligament, Conoid ligament
- Supraspinatus muscle
- Middle glenohumeral ligament
- Anterior inferior glenohumeral ligament

Rotator Cuff Tear

- Supraspinatus muscle tendon fixed with stitches
- Tear in supraspinatus muscle tendon

Lateral View

Acromioplasty

Acromioplasty is a type of surgery done to surgically remove the coracoacromial ligament (**a**) and the anterior lip and underside of the acromion (shaded gray) (**b**).

The rotator cuff is made up of the tendons from the subscapularis, the supraspinatus, the infraspinatus, and the teres minor muscles. Tearing of these tendons, which are primarily responsible for shoulder joint motion, can result from trauma or chronic impingement. Surgical repair may be necessary to restore function.

Neutral
- Subacromial bursa
- Acromion
- Supraspinatus tendon & muscle
- Greater tuberosity

Abduction
- Compression point

Impingement Syndrome

Impingement syndrome is one of the most common shoulder problems. When the arm is abducted past 90°, the greater tuberosity of the humerus compresses the rotator cuff against the acromion causing pain and decreased motion in the shoulder.

Acromioclavicular Separation
- Acromioclavicular ligament
- Trapezoid ligament (torn)
- Conoid ligament (torn)

Grade I — Grade II — Grade III

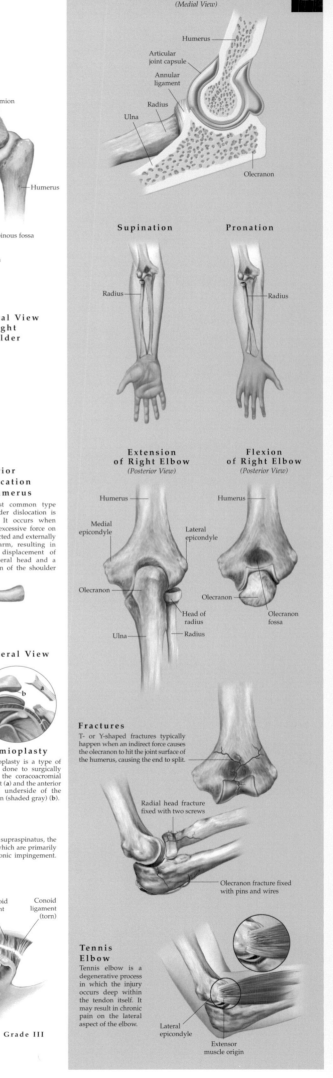

Sagittal Section of Right Elbow *(Medial View)*
- Humerus
- Articular joint capsule
- Annular ligament
- Radius
- Ulna
- Olecranon

Supination
- Radius

Pronation
- Radius

Extension of Right Elbow *(Posterior View)*
- Humerus
- Medial epicondyle
- Olecranon
- Ulna
- Head of radius
- Radius

Flexion of Right Elbow *(Posterior View)*
- Humerus
- Lateral epicondyle
- Olecranon
- Olecranon fossa

Fractures

T- or Y-shaped fractures typically happen when an indirect force causes the olecranon to hit the joint surface of the humerus, causing the end to split.

Radial head fracture fixed with two screws

Olecranon fracture fixed with pins and wires

Tennis Elbow

Tennis elbow is a degenerative process in which the injury occurs deep within the tendon itself. It may result in chronic pain on the lateral aspect of the elbow.
- Lateral epicondyle
- Extensor muscle origin

©2008 Wolters Kluwer Health | Lippincott Williams & Wilkins | Published by Anatomical Chart Company, Skokie, IL

The Skin and Common Disorders

Normal Anatomy

The skin is the body's largest organ. It covers the entire body and weighs approximately six pounds. The skin includes two primary layers: the outer epidermis and the inner dermis. The epidermis has important protective functions. It protects against injury and excessive water loss. It also prevents disease-causing microorganisms from entering the body.

The thick dermis contains blood vessels, nerve endings, and glands that respond to heat, pressure, and pain. Beneath the dermis, the subcutaneous layer is made up of loose connective tissue and fat (adipose) tissue. This layer acts as a cushion for the skin, helps maintain body heat, and is a store of energy.

Derivatives of Skin

Derivatives of skin include hair, sebaceous glands, sweat glands and nails. These structures all derive from specialized areas of the epidermis that grow down into the dermis.

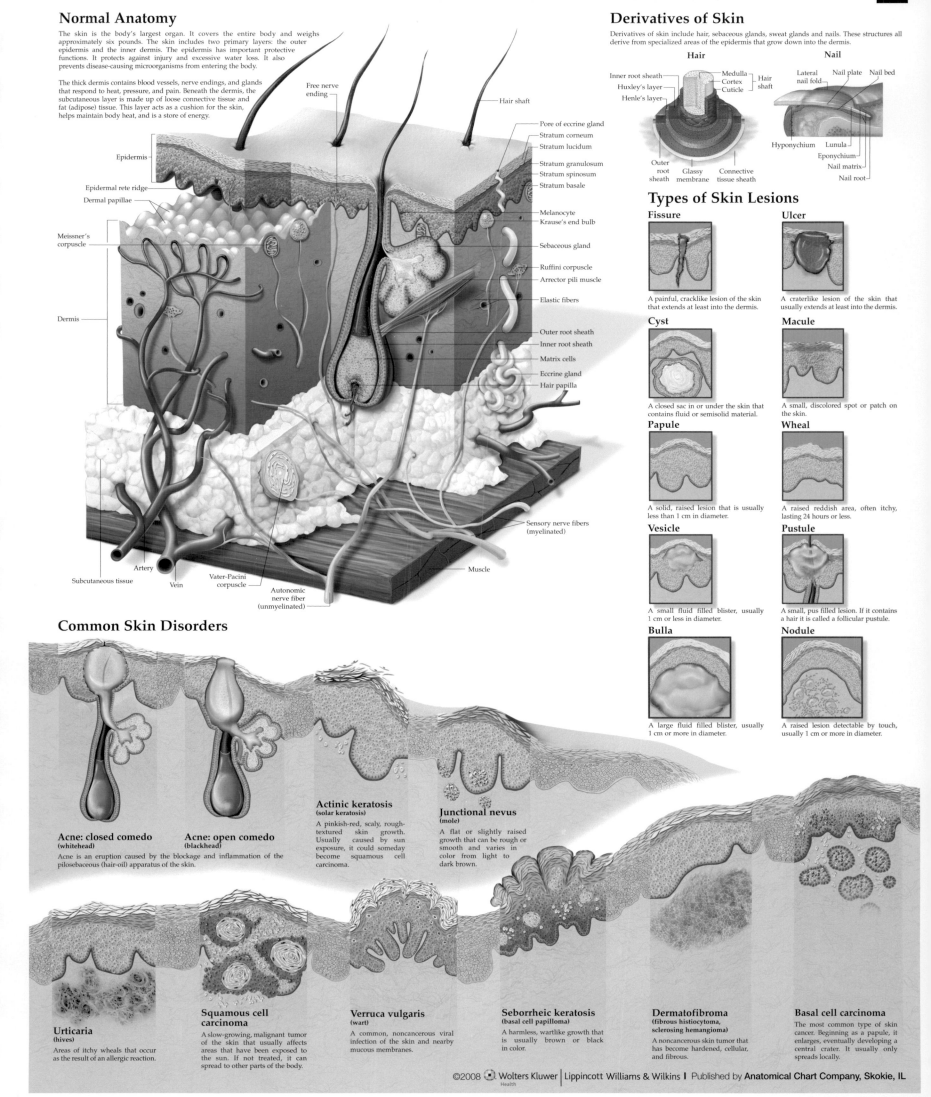

Hair

Inner root sheath
Huxley's layer
Henle's layer
Medulla
Cortex
Cuticle
Hair shaft
Outer root sheath
Glassy membrane
Connective tissue sheath

Nail

Lateral nail fold
Nail plate
Nail bed
Hyponychium
Lunula
Eponychium
Nail matrix
Nail root

Normal Anatomy labels

Free nerve ending
Hair shaft
Pore of eccrine gland
Stratum corneum
Stratum lucidum
Stratum granulosum
Stratum spinosum
Stratum basale
Epidermis
Epidermal rete ridge
Dermal papillae
Melanocyte
Krause's end bulb
Sebaceous gland
Ruffini corpuscle
Arrector pili muscle
Elastic fibers
Meissner's corpuscle
Dermis
Outer root sheath
Inner root sheath
Matrix cells
Eccrine gland
Hair papilla
Sensory nerve fibers (myelinated)
Subcutaneous tissue
Artery
Vein
Vater-Pacini corpuscle
Autonomic nerve fiber (unmyelinated)
Muscle

Types of Skin Lesions

Fissure
A painful, cracklike lesion of the skin that extends at least into the dermis.

Ulcer
A craterlike lesion of the skin that usually extends at least into the dermis.

Cyst
A closed sac in or under the skin that contains fluid or semisolid material.

Macule
A small, discolored spot or patch on the skin.

Papule
A solid, raised lesion that is usually less than 1 cm in diameter.

Wheal
A raised reddish area, often itchy, lasting 24 hours or less.

Vesicle
A small fluid filled blister, usually 1 cm or less in diameter.

Pustule
A small, pus filled lesion. If it contains a hair it is called a follicular pustule.

Bulla
A large fluid filled blister, usually 1 cm or more in diameter.

Nodule
A raised lesion detectable by touch, usually 1 cm or more in diameter.

Common Skin Disorders

Acne: closed comedo (whitehead)

Acne: open comedo (blackhead)
Acne is an eruption caused by the blockage and inflammation of the pilosebaceous (hair-oil) apparatus of the skin.

Actinic keratosis (solar keratosis)
A pinkish-red, scaly, rough-textured skin growth. Usually caused by sun exposure, it could someday become squamous cell carcinoma.

Junctional nevus (mole)
A flat or slightly raised growth that can be rough or smooth and varies in color from light to dark brown.

Urticaria (hives)
Areas of itchy wheals that occur as the result of an allergic reaction.

Squamous cell carcinoma
A slow-growing, malignant tumor of the skin that usually affects areas that have been exposed to the sun. If not treated, it can spread to other parts of the body.

Verruca vulgaris (wart)
A common, noncancerous viral infection of the skin and nearby mucous membranes.

Seborrheic keratosis (basal cell papilloma)
A harmless, wartlike growth that is usually brown or black in color.

Dermatofibroma (fibrous histiocytoma, sclerosing hemangioma)
A noncancerous skin tumor that has become hardened, cellular, and fibrous.

Basal cell carcinoma
The most common type of skin cancer. Beginning as a papule, it enlarges, eventually developing a central crater. It usually only spreads locally.

©2008 Wolters Kluwer Health | Lippincott Williams & Wilkins | Published by Anatomical Chart Company, Skokie, IL

The Human Skull

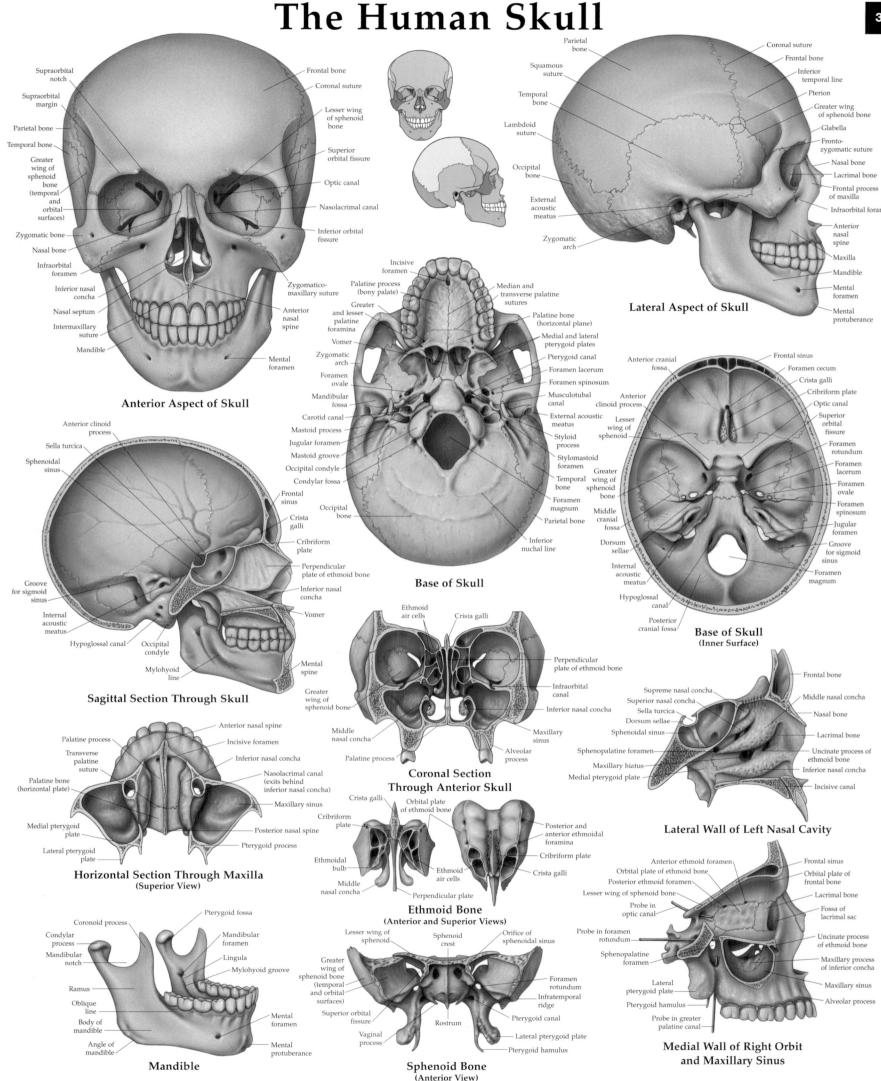

Anterior Aspect of Skull

Lateral Aspect of Skull

Sagittal Section Through Skull

Base of Skull

Base of Skull
(Inner Surface)

Horizontal Section Through Maxilla
(Superior View)

Coronal Section
Through Anterior Skull

Lateral Wall of Left Nasal Cavity

Ethmoid Bone
(Anterior and Superior Views)

Mandible

Sphenoid Bone
(Anterior View)

Medial Wall of Right Orbit
and Maxillary Sinus

©2008 Wolters Kluwer | Lippincott Williams & Wilkins I Published by Anatomical Chart Company, Skokie, IL
Health

Anatomy of the Teeth

Primary Teeth

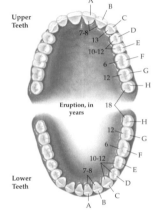

Upper Teeth

A
B
C
F
G
6
7-8
16
12
24

Eruption, in months

Lower Teeth

24
12
16
6
7-8
C
A B
F
G

Permanent Teeth

Upper Teeth

A
B
C
D
E
F
G
H
7-8
13
10-12
6
12

Eruption, in years

18

Lower Teeth

H
G
F
E
D
C
B
A
12
6
10-12
7-8

A Central incisor
B Lateral incisor
C Canine
D First premolar
E Second premolar
F First molar
G Second molar
H Third molar

Function of the Teeth

Incisor: Acts like scissors; grasps and cuts food.

Bicuspid: Has two pointed projections; tears, shreds, crushes food.

Cuspid: Has a single, very long, sharp cusp; tears and shreds food.

Molar: Strongest, most useful type of tooth; grinds food into tiny pieces.

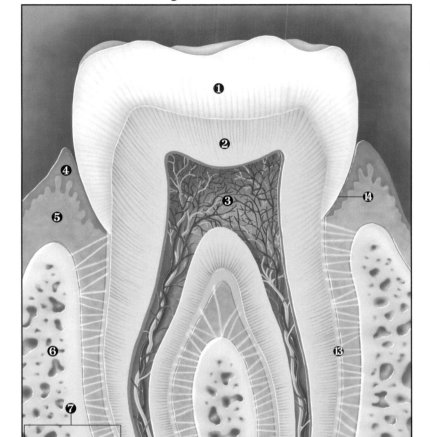

1 Enamel
2 Dentin, with dentinal tubules
3 Pulp chamber containing vessels and nerves
4 Gingival (gum) epithelium
5 Lamina propria of gingiva (gum)
6 Bone
7 Periodontium
8 Periodontal membranes
9 Root canal
10 Interradicular septum
11 Apical foramina
12 Odontoblast layer
13 Cementum
14 Gingival sulcus

Childhood Dentition

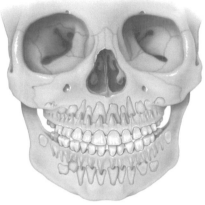

Beneath the erupted primary (baby or milk) teeth lie the permanent teeth (shown in blue). The twenty primary teeth are replaced as the child grows. Eruption and shedding dates are shown in the drawings on the far left.

Oral Cavity

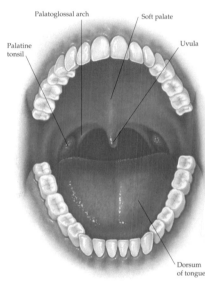

Palatoglossal arch
Soft palate
Palatine tonsil
Uvula
Dorsum of tongue

Tooth Decay

1 Decay of enamel
2 Decay invades dentin
3 Inflammation of pulp
4 Death of pulp
5 Abscess formation

Innervation and Blood Supply

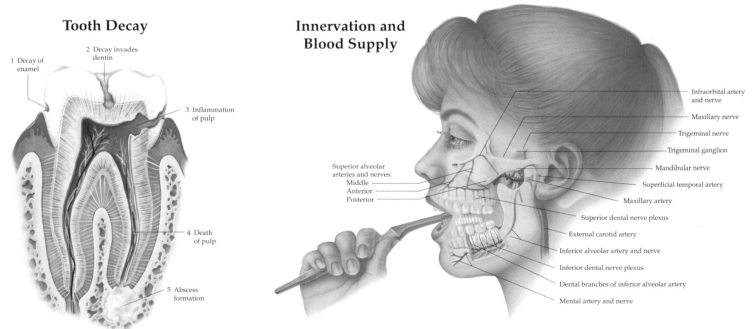

Infraorbital artery and nerve
Maxillary nerve
Trigeminal nerve
Trigeminal ganglion
Mandibular nerve
Superficial temporal artery
Maxillary artery
Superior dental nerve plexus
External carotid artery
Inferior alveolar artery and nerve
Inferior dental nerve plexus
Dental branches of inferior alveolar artery
Mental artery and nerve

Superior alveolar arteries and nerves:
Middle
Anterior
Posterior

The Vertebral Column

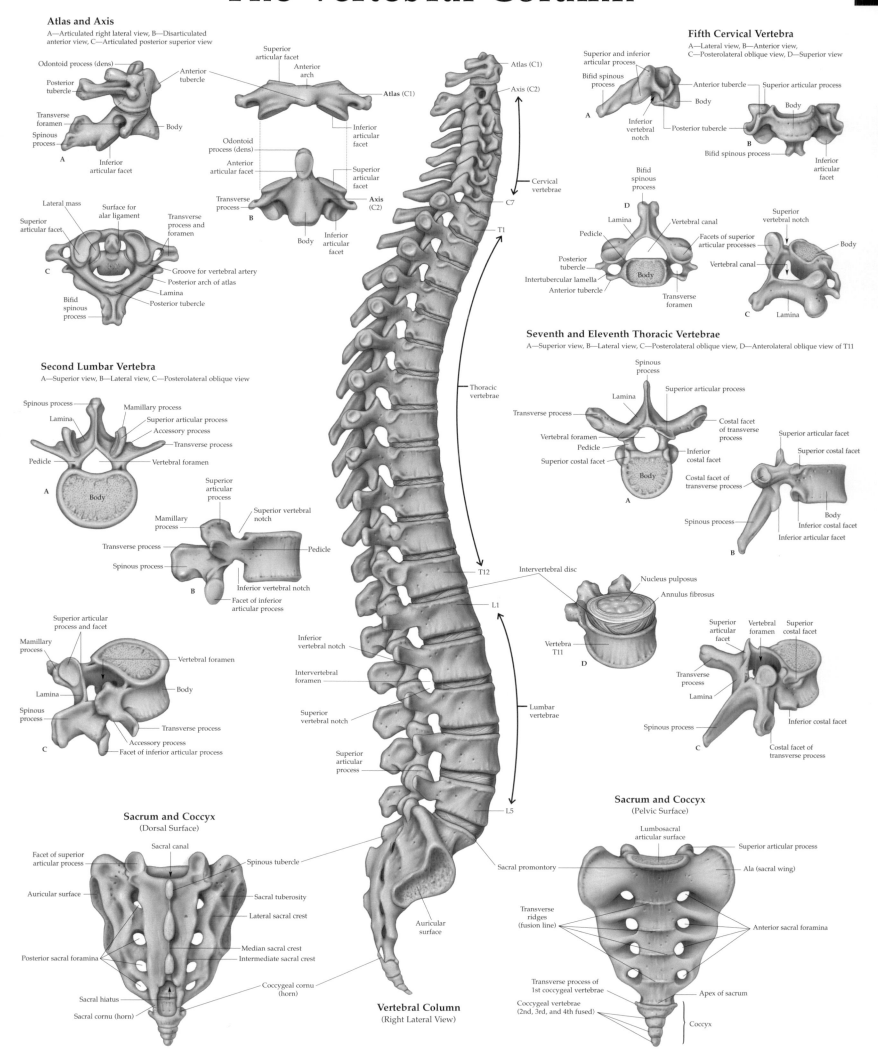

Atlas and Axis
A—Articulated right lateral view, B—Disarticulated anterior view, C—Articulated posterior superior view

Odontoid process (dens)
Posterior tubercle
Transverse foramen
Spinous process
Anterior tubercle
Body
Inferior articular facet
A

Superior articular facet
Anterior arch
Atlas (C1)
Inferior articular facet
Odontoid process (dens)
Anterior articular facet
Transverse process
Superior articular facet
Axis (C2)
Body
Inferior articular facet
B

Lateral mass
Surface for alar ligament
Superior articular facet
Transverse process and foramen
Groove for vertebral artery
Posterior arch of atlas
Lamina
Posterior tubercle
Bifid spinous process
C

Fifth Cervical Vertebra
A—Lateral view, B—Anterior view, C—Posterolateral oblique view, D—Superior view

Superior and inferior articular process
Bifid spinous process
Anterior tubercle
Body
Inferior vertebral notch
Posterior tubercle
A

Superior articular process
Body
Bifid spinous process
Inferior articular facet
B

Bifid spinous process
Lamina
Pedicle
Posterior tubercle
Intertubercular lamella
Anterior tubercle
Vertebral canal
Facets of superior articular processes
Body
Transverse foramen
D

Superior vertebral notch
Body
Vertebral canal
Lamina
C

Atlas (C1)
Axis (C2)
Cervical vertebrae
C7
T1

Second Lumbar Vertebra
A—Superior view, B—Lateral view, C—Posterolateral oblique view

Spinous process
Lamina
Pedicle
Mamillary process
Superior articular process
Accessory process
Transverse process
Vertebral foramen
Body
A

Superior articular process
Superior vertebral notch
Mamillary process
Transverse process
Spinous process
Pedicle
Inferior vertebral notch
Facet of inferior articular process
B

Superior articular process and facet
Mamillary process
Vertebral foramen
Lamina
Spinous process
Body
Transverse process
Accessory process
Facet of inferior articular process
C

Thoracic vertebrae
T12
L1

Seventh and Eleventh Thoracic Vertebrae
A—Superior view, B—Lateral view, C—Posterolateral oblique view, D—Anterolateral oblique view of T11

Spinous process
Lamina
Transverse process
Vertebral foramen
Pedicle
Superior costal facet
Superior articular process
Costal facet of transverse process
Inferior costal facet
Body
A

Superior articular facet
Superior costal facet
Costal facet of transverse process
Body
Inferior costal facet
Inferior articular facet
Spinous process
B

Intervertebral disc
Nucleus pulposus
Annulus fibrosus
Vertebra T11
D

Superior articular facet
Vertebral foramen
Superior costal facet
Transverse process
Lamina
Spinous process
Inferior costal facet
Costal facet of transverse process
C

Intervertebral foramen
Inferior vertebral notch
Superior vertebral notch
Superior articular process
Lumbar vertebrae
L5

Sacrum and Coccyx
(Dorsal Surface)

Sacral canal
Facet of superior articular process
Auricular surface
Spinous tubercle
Sacral tuberosity
Lateral sacral crest
Posterior sacral foramina
Median sacral crest
Intermediate sacral crest
Coccygeal cornu (horn)
Sacral hiatus
Sacral cornu (horn)

Vertebral Column
(Right Lateral View)

Sacral promontory
Auricular surface

Sacrum and Coccyx
(Pelvic Surface)

Lumbosacral articular surface
Superior articular process
Sacral promontory
Ala (sacral wing)
Transverse ridges (fusion line)
Anterior sacral foramina
Transverse process of 1st coccygeal vertebrae
Apex of sacrum
Coccygeal vertebrae (2nd, 3rd, and 4th fused)
Coccyx

©2008 Wolters Kluwer Health | Lippincott Williams & Wilkins | Published by Anatomical Chart Company, Skokie, IL

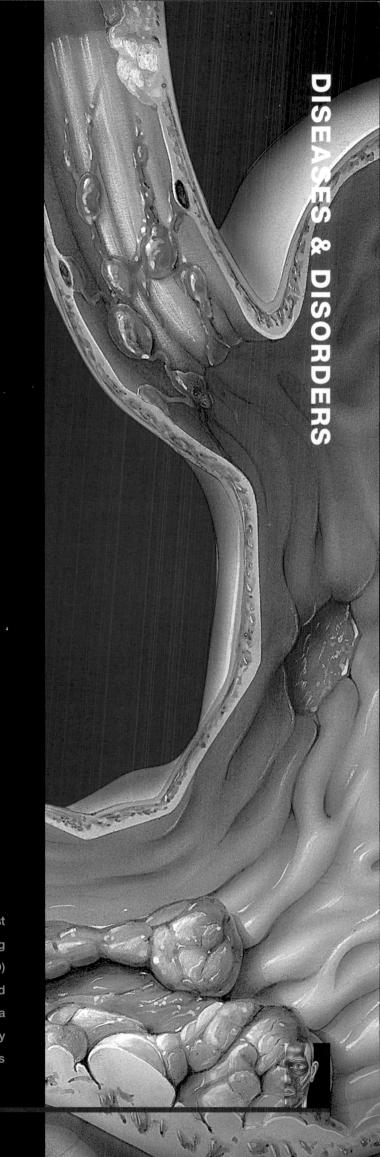

What Is An Allergy?

An allergy is an overreaction or hypersensitivity of the body's immune system to normally harmless substances, called allergens. An allergic reaction occurs when the body's immune system responds to an allergen as if the substance were disease causing. Subsequent exposures to this substance can result in physical symptoms that range from mild to life threatening.

Who Gets Allergies?

The tendency to develop allergies is thought to be inherited, because they commonly develop in those who have a family history of allergies. It is possible for anyone to develop allergies at any age. Environmental factors can make our immune systems overly sensitive. This could then trigger allergies in people with no family history or hasten the onset in those with a family history.

What Are Common Allergens?

Allergens can enter the body in a number of different ways, including inhaling, eating/drinking, injection (as with bee venom), and contact with the skin or eyes. Common allergens include pollen, mold, animal hair or dander, dust mites, certain medications (for example, penicillin), and certain foods (for example, peanuts, eggs, milk, wheat, and seafood).

Anaphylaxis: An Allergic Emergency

Anaphylaxis is a life-threatening reaction. The onset of this reaction may occur within seconds or minutes of exposure. Symptoms may include a red rash over most of the body. Skin becomes warm to the touch, intense tightening and swelling of the airways make breathing difficult, and there is a drop in blood pressure. Breathing can stop and the body may slip into shock. If medication is not administered quickly, heart failure and death can result within minutes in the most severe reactions. Allergens in insect venom and medications such as antibiotics are more likely to cause anaphylaxis than are any other allergens. Anaphylaxis is not a common reaction and can be controlled with prompt medication and the help of a physician.

Managing Allergies

The first step in managing allergies is to identify the type of reaction you are having, whether it is watery eyes, sneezing, or difficulty breathing. Second, try to identify the trigger or the situation that led to the symptoms. Ask yourself a few questions:

- *Where did the reaction occur?*
- *Inside or outside?*
- *Were you eating or drinking?*
- *Were there any animals or insects near you?*
- *Were you wearing any new clothing?*
- *Did you use a new soap or detergent?*

A physician can perform skin or blood allergy tests with a variety of common allergens. Once the allergen has been identified, manage your allergies by following some tips:

- *Avoid allergens when possible.*
- *Avoid tobacco smoke and other irritants.*
- *Use medication as prescribed.*
- *See a doctor regularly.*
- *Stay healthy.*

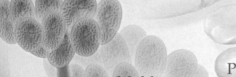

Seafood

Drugs

Mold

Peanuts

Pollen

Dander Dust mites

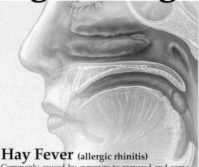

Hay Fever (allergic rhinitis)

Commonly caused by exposure to ragweed and some tree pollens. It affects the eyes and nose. Causes sneezing; runny nose; watery, itchy eyes; irritated, itchy throat; and sometimes, a stuffy, blocked nose.

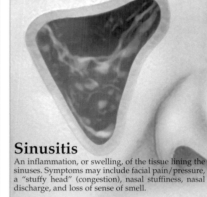

Sinusitis

An inflammation, or swelling, of the tissue lining the sinuses. Symptoms may include facial pain/pressure, a "stuffy head" (congestion), nasal stuffiness, nasal discharge, and loss of sense of smell.

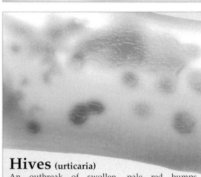

Eczema (atopic dermatitis)

A group of medical conditions that cause the skin to become inflamed or irritated. It causes itchy, red rashes of the skin characterized by lesions, scaling, and flaking.

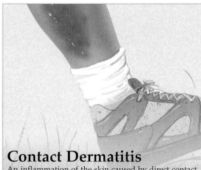

Hives (urticaria)

An outbreak of swollen, pale red bumps or patches (wheals) on the skin, as a result of the body's adverse reaction to certain allergens, or for unknown reasons.

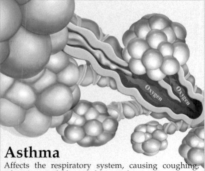

Asthma

Affects the respiratory system, causing coughing, wheezing, and chest tightness after exposure to an allergen. Common allergens that worsen asthma include plant pollens and dust mites.

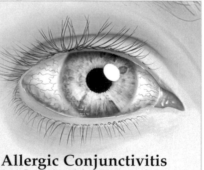

Contact Dermatitis

An inflammation of the skin caused by direct contact with an irritating or allergy-causing substance (such as poison ivy or latex gloves). It causes redness, itching, swelling, or rashes on the skin.

Allergic Conjunctivitis

An inflammation of the conjunctiva, the tissue that lines the eyeball and inside of the eyelid, associated with allergies. The eye becomes red, itchy, and watery.

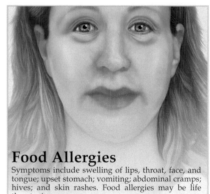

Food Allergies

Symptoms include swelling of lips, throat, face, and tongue; upset stomach; vomiting; abdominal cramps; hives; and skin rashes. Food allergies may be life threatening.

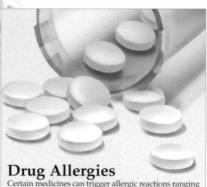

Drug Allergies

Certain medicines can trigger allergic reactions ranging from mild rashes to life-threatening symptoms, which can affect any tissue or organ in the body.

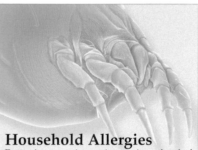

Household Allergies

Dust mites are microscopic organisms that feed on live and shed skin tissue. Mites are commonly found on pillows, mattresses, and upholstered furniture. Mite feces are responsible for a majority of the year-round types of allergies, and are a major cause of asthma.

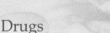

©2008 Wolters Kluwer Health | Lippincott Williams & Wilkins | Published by Anatomical Chart Company, Skokie, IL

Understanding Arthritis

Osteoarthritis (OA)

- Most common type of arthritis.
- Primarily affects cartilage, the tissue that cushions the ends of bones within the joints.
- May initially affect joints asymmetrically.
- Affects hands and weight bearing joints.
- Can cause joint pain and stiffness.
- Usually develops slowly over many years.

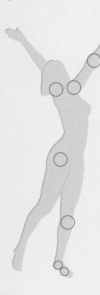

○ = identifies areas most affected by OA.

Rheumatoid Arthritis (RA)

- Causes redness, warmth, and swelling of joints.
- Usually affects the same joint on both sides of the body.
- Often causes a general feeling of sickness, fatigue, weight loss, and fever.
- May develop suddenly, within weeks or months.
- Most often begins between ages 25 and 50.

○ = identifies areas most affected by RA.

Other Arthritic Diseases

Many people use the word *arthritis* to refer to all rheumatic diseases. However, the word literally means joint inflammation. Other types of arthritis include:

Fibromyalgia (Fibrositis)

- Chronic disorder that causes pain throughout the tissues that support and move the bones and joints.
- Pain, stiffness, and localized tender points occur in the muscles and tendons, particularly those of the spine, shoulders, and hips.
- Patients may also experience fatigue and sleep disturbances.

Gout

- Results from deposits of needle-like crystals of uric acid in the joints.
- The crystals cause inflammation, swelling, and pain in the affected joint, which is often the big toe.

Juvenile Rheumatoid Arthritis

- Most common form of arthritis in children.
- Causes pain, stiffness, swelling, and impaired function of the joints.
- May be associated with rashes or fevers; may affect various parts of the body.

Systemic Lupus Erythematosus

- Also known as *lupus* or *SLE*.
- Can result in inflammation of and damage to the joints, skin, kidneys, heart, lungs, blood vessels, and brain.

Bursitis

- Inflammation of a bursa, a small, fluid-filled sac that absorbs shock and reduces friction around a joint.
- May be caused by arthritis in the joint or by injury or infection of the bursa.
- Produces pain and tenderness and may limit the movement of nearby joints.

Tendinitis

- Inflammation of a tendon, a cord of fibrous tissue that attaches muscle to bone.
- May be caused by overuse, injury, or a rheumatic condition.
- Produces pain and tenderness and may restrict movement of nearby joints.

Common Symptoms of Arthritis

- Swelling in one or more joints.
- Stiffness around the joints (each episode of stiffness for RA lasts one hour or more, but OA lasts 30 minutes or less).
- Constant or recurring pain or tenderness in a joint.
- Difficulty using or moving a joint normally.
- Warmth and redness in a joint.

If you have any of these symptoms for more than two weeks, contact your physician.

Joints Affected by Osteoarthritis (OA)

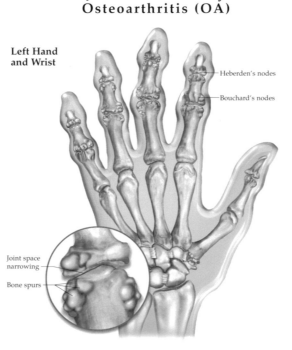

Left Hand and Wrist — Heberden's nodes, Bouchard's nodes, Joint space narrowing, Bone spurs

Joints Affected by Rheumatoid Arthritis (RA)

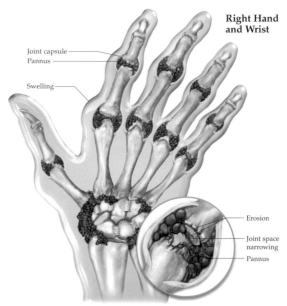

Right Hand and Wrist — Joint capsule, Pannus, Swelling, Erosion, Joint space narrowing, Pannus

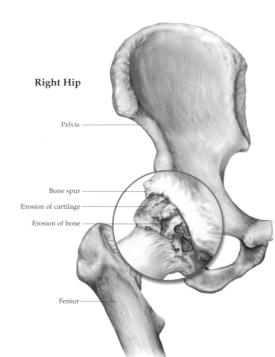

Right Hip — Pelvis, Bone spur, Erosion of cartilage, Erosion of bone, Femur

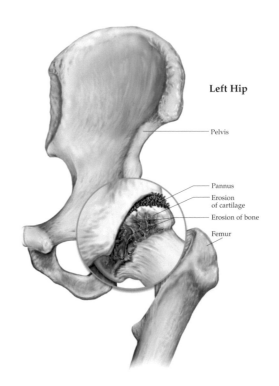

Left Hip — Pelvis, Pannus, Erosion of cartilage, Erosion of bone, Femur

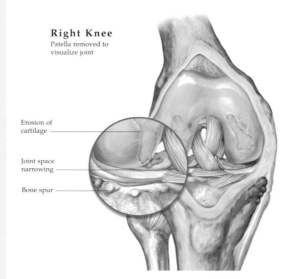

Right Knee — Patella removed to visualize joint — Erosion of cartilage, Joint space narrowing, Bone spur

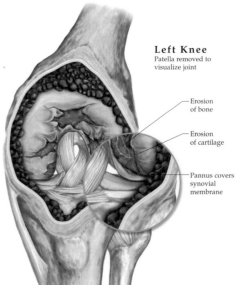

Left Knee — Patella removed to visualize joint — Erosion of bone, Erosion of cartilage, Pannus covers synovial membrane

Understanding Asthma

Carbon dioxide exhaled

Oxygen inhaled

What Happens in an Asthma Attack?

What Is Asthma?

Asthma is a chronic disease of the lungs in which inflammation causes the airways to narrow, making breathing more difficult.

What Causes Asthma?

Although the actual cause of asthma is not known, many studies have shown that it may be due to a combination of factors. We do know that asthma is not contagious like the flu. We also know that people have a higher risk of developing asthma if a family member has had an asthma attack or if they live with people who smoke.

How Is Asthma Diagnosed?

There is no single or definitive test for asthma. It is diagnosed based on a review of the patient's medical history and those of his or her family. There are many tests your doctor may use to get more information about your condition. These include pulmonary function tests, allergy tests, blood tests, and chest and sinus x-rays.

A Smooth muscle tightens the airways.

Smooth muscle

Alveoli

How Do the Lungs Work?

When you breathe, you draw in (inhale) fresh air and oxygen into your lungs and expel (exhale) stale air and carbon dioxide from your lungs.

1. The incoming air goes through a network of airways (bronchial tubes) that reach the lungs.

2. As the air moves through the lungs, the bronchial tubes become progressively smaller, like branches of a tree.

3. At the end of the smallest tubes are alveolar sacs, the site of gas exchange between the lungs and the circulatory system.

4. Oxygen enters the alveolar sacs, where it passes to the bloodstream and is then used by the body.

5. Carbon dioxide (waste product) from the bloodstream enters the alveolar sacs to be carried out of the lungs.

B Sides of airways have become inflamed and swollen, making it harder for oxygen to get to alveoli.

Oxygen

C Excess mucus has formed inside the airways.

Sides of airways are thin to allow more space for oxygen to get to alveoli.

Oxygen

Monitoring Your Asthma by Zone

Green Zone	Yellow Zone	Red Zone
No asthma symptoms. Able to do usual activities and sleep without coughing, wheezing, or breathing difficulty.	There may be coughing, wheezing, and mild shortness of breath. Sleep and usual activities may be disturbed. May be more tired than usual.	Symptoms may include frequent, severe cough; severe shortness of breath; wheezing; trouble talking while walking; rapid breathing.
Action: Keep controlling/preventing your asthma symptoms. Continue to take your asthma medicines exactly as prescribed by your healthcare specialist, even if you have no symptoms and feel fine.	**Action:** Keep controlling your asthma symptoms and add your prescribed quick-relief medicine. Call to discuss the situation with your doctor or healthcare specialist.	**Action:** Go to an emergency room.

Bronchiole During an Asthma Attack

Symptoms of Asthma

Symptoms of asthma often vary from time to time in an individual. The severity of an asthma attack can increase rapidly, so it is important to treat your symptoms immediately once you recognize them.

Adult Symptoms
• Wheezing
• Chest tightness
• Coughing
• Difficulty breathing: shortness of breath

Childhood Symptoms
• Coughing at night or during sleep
• Diminished responsiveness
• Constant rattly cough
• Frequent chest colds
• Rapid breathing
• Weak cry
• Grunt when nursing or have difficulty feeding
• Chest might feel "funny"
• Unexplained irritability

Common Asthma Triggers

The airways in an asthmatic person are extremely sensitive to certain factors known as triggers. When stimulated by these triggers, the airways overreact with abnormal inflammation that leads to swelling, increased mucus secretion, and muscle contraction of the air passages. Examples of asthma triggers include:

• Pollution: cigarette smoke,* smog, strong odors from painting or cooking, scented products
• Allergens: animal dander, dust mites, cockroaches, pollen, mold
• Cold air or changes in weather
• Illness and infections
• Exercise
• Medications such as pain relievers
• Sulfites or other additives in food and beverages
• GERD (gastroesophageal reflux disease)

The proteins on dust mites are among the allergens that may trigger an asthma attack.

People can have trouble with one or more triggers. Your doctor can help you identify your asthma triggers and ways to avoid them.

*The risk of asthma is increased in children who are regularly exposed to cigarette smoke.

Management of Asthma

Asthma is a chronic disease that can be controlled to allow normal daily activities. By controlling your asthma every day, you can prevent serious symptoms and take part in all activities. If your asthma is not well controlled, you are likely to have symptoms that can make you miss school or work and keep you from doing other things you enjoy. Although there is no cure, here are some important prevention strategies:

• Recognize attacks early.
• Take medication as directed.
• Avoid tobacco smoke.
• Identify and avoid triggers.
• Talk with your doctor to find ways to improve your health.
• Get the influenza vaccination (flu shot) every year and a pneumococcal vaccination (pneumonia shot) every five years.

Healthy Bronchiole

©2008 Wolters Kluwer Health | Lippincott Williams & Wilkins | Published by Anatomical Chart Company, Skokie, IL

Understanding Breast Cancer

What Is Breast Cancer?

Breast cancer is the most common form of cancer in women and is the number two killer (after lung cancer) of women age 35 to 54. It can also occur in men, though incidence is rare. The survival rate has improved because of earlier diagnosis and the variety of treatments now available. Most breast cancer occurs in the upper outer quadrant (the upper part of the breast closest to the arm). A woman may not be able to feel a slow-growing breast tumor by touch for up to eight years, until it is 1-centimeter in diameter. Breast cancer may spread by way of the lymphatic system or bloodstream to the lungs, liver, bones and other organs, or directly to the skin or surrounding tissues.

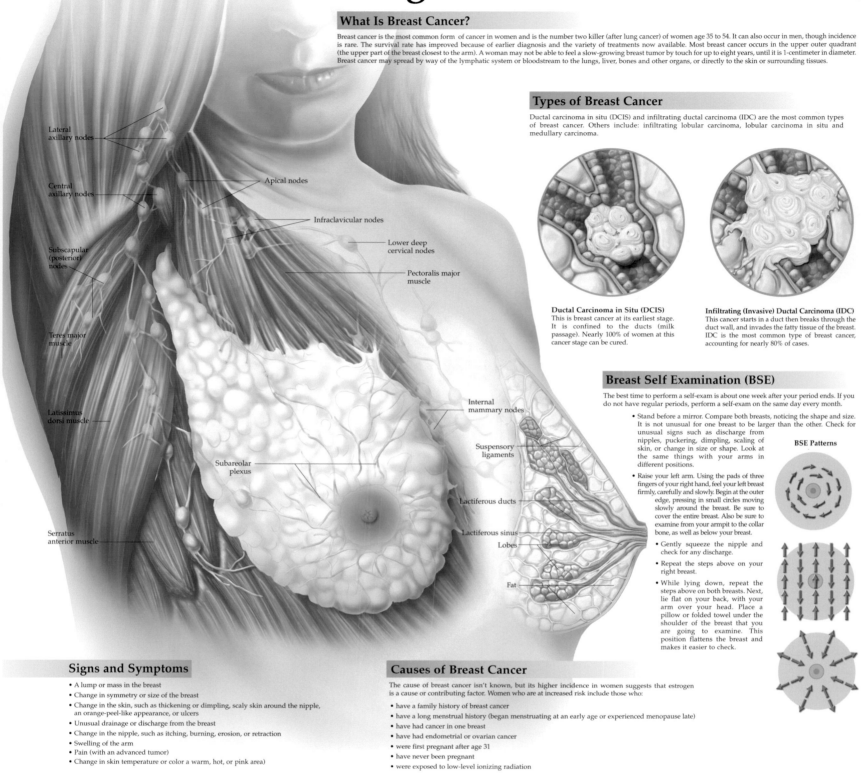

Types of Breast Cancer

Ductal carcinoma in situ (DCIS) and infiltrating ductal carcinoma (IDC) are the most common types of breast cancer. Others include: infiltrating lobular carcinoma, lobular carcinoma in situ and medullary carcinoma.

Ductal Carcinoma in Situ (DCIS)
This is breast cancer at its earliest stage. It is confined to the ducts (milk passage). Nearly 100% of women at this cancer stage can be cured.

Infiltrating (Invasive) Ductal Carcinoma (IDC)
This cancer starts in a duct then breaks through the duct wall, and invades the fatty tissue of the breast. IDC is the most common type of breast cancer, accounting for nearly 80% of cases.

Breast Self Examination (BSE)

The best time to perform a self-exam is about one week after your period ends. If you do not have regular periods, perform a self-exam on the same day every month.

- Stand before a mirror. Compare both breasts, noticing the shape and size. It is not unusual for one breast to be larger than the other. Check for unusual signs such as discharge from nipples, puckering, dimpling, scaling of skin, or change in size or shape. Look at the same things with your arms in different positions.
- Raise your left arm. Using the pads of three fingers of your right hand, feel your left breast firmly, carefully and slowly. Begin at the outer edge, pressing in small circles moving slowly around the breast. Be sure to cover the entire breast. Also be sure to examine from your armpit to the collar bone, as well as below your breast.
- Gently squeeze the nipple and check for any discharge.
- Repeat the steps above on your right breast.
- While lying down, repeat the steps above on both breasts. Next, lie flat on your back, with your arm over your head. Place a pillow or folded towel under the shoulder of the breast that you are going to examine. This position flattens the breast and makes it easier to check.

BSE Patterns

Signs and Symptoms

- A lump or mass in the breast
- Change in symmetry or size of the breast
- Change in the skin, such as thickening or dimpling, scaly skin around the nipple, an orange-peel-like appearance, or ulcers
- Unusual drainage or discharge from the breast
- Change in the nipple, such as itching, burning, erosion, or retraction
- Swelling of the arm
- Pain (with an advanced tumor)
- Change in skin temperature or color a warm, hot, or pink area)

Causes of Breast Cancer

The cause of breast cancer isn't known, but its higher incidence in women suggests that estrogen is a cause or contributing factor. Women who are at increased risk include those who:

- have a family history of breast cancer
- have a long menstrual history (began menstruating at an early age or experienced menopause late)
- have had cancer in one breast
- have had endometrial or ovarian cancer
- were first pregnant after age 31
- have never been pregnant
- were exposed to low-level ionizing radiation

Staging

Clinical staging is a part of the pretreatment evaluation and is performed by histologic examination of the biopsied tissue and axillary specimen to assess the extent of the disease, lymph node involvement, the status of the other breast, and the possibility of systemic metastasis (passing from one site to another).
The most commonly used system is the **Tumor-Nodes-Metastasis system (TNM)**. **T** represents the primary tumor, **N** describes lymph node involvement, and **M** describes metastasis, if any.

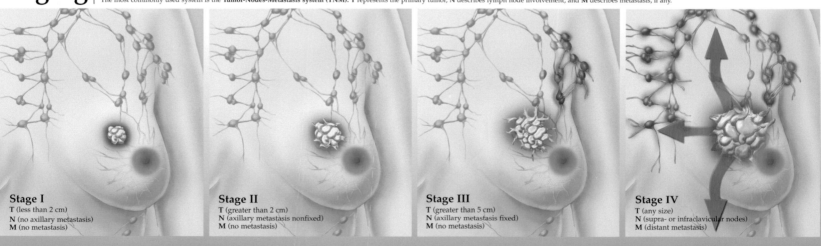

Stage I
T (less than 2 cm)
N (no axillary metastasis)
M (no metastasis)

Stage II
T (greater than 2 cm)
N (axillary metastasis nonfixed)
M (no metastasis)

Stage III
T (greater than 5 cm)
N (axillary metastasis fixed)
M (no metastasis)

Stage IV
T (any size)
N (supra- or infraclavicular nodes)
M (distant metastasis)

Understanding Colorectal Cancer

Transverse colon

Adenocarcinoma of colon

Circumferencial carcinoma of transverse colon

Ascending colon

Cecum

Colonic polyps

Adenocarcinoma of jejunum

Vermiform appendix

Descending colon

Adenocarcinoma of rectosigmoid region

Rectum

Anus

Sigmoid colon

What is Colorectal Cancer? Cancer that begins in the colon is called colon cancer and cancer that begins in the rectum is called rectal cancer. Cancers affecting either of these organs is also called colorectal cancer.

Colorectal cancer occurs when some of the cells that line the colon or the rectum become abnormal and grow out of control. The abnormal growing cells create a tumor, which is the cancer.

Who is at Risk for Colorectal Cancer? Everybody is at risk for colorectal cancer. Colorectal cancer is the 2nd leading type of cancer causing deaths in the U.S.A. The majority of people who develop colorectal cancer have no known risk factors.

The exact cause of colorectal cancer is not yet known. Below are some factors that could increase a person's risk of developing this disease.

- **Age** - The disease is more common in people over 50. The chance of getting colorectal cancer increases with each decade of life. However, it has also been detected in younger people.
- **Gender** - Overall the risks are equal, but women have a higher risk for colon cancer and men are more likely to develop rectal cancer.
- **Polyps** - Begin as non-cancerous growths on the inner wall of the colon or rectum; this is fairly common in people over 50 years of age. Adenomas are one type of non-cancerous polyps that can mutate and are the potential precursors of colon and rectal cancer.
- **Personal history** - Research shows that women who have a history of ovarian or uterine cancer have a slight increased risk of developing colorectal cancer. In addition, people who have Ulcerative colitis or Crohn's disease also are at higher risk.
- **Family history** - Parents, siblings, and children of a person who has had colorectal cancer are more likely to develop the disease themselves. A family history of familial polyposis, adenomatous polyps, or hereditary polyp syndrome also increases the risk.
- **Diet** - A diet high in fat and calories and low in fiber may be linked to a greater risk.
- **Lifestyle factors** - Alcohol, smoking, lack of exercise, and overweight status are additional risk factors.
- **Diabetes** - Diabetics have a 30-40% increased risk.

Signs & Symptoms

Colorectal cancer may not cause any symptoms in early stages. However the following signs should raise suspicion:

- Change in bowel habits: Diarrhea or constipation or a change in the consistency of stool
- Narrow, pencil-thin stools
- Rectal bleed or blood in stool
- Persistent abdominal discomfort such as gas, pain or cramps
- Feeling bowel does not empty completely
- Unexplained weight loss
- Constant fatigue

Screening tests

- **Fecal Occult Blood Test (FOBT)** - Checks for hidden blood in the stool.
- **Sigmoidoscopy** - Sigmoidoscope is a long, flexible tube with a tiny video camera at the tip that is inserted into the rectum to allow the doctor to view the lower part of the colon – the rectum, the descending colon, and the sigmoid colon.
- **Colonoscopy** - Colonoscope is a long, flexible tube with a tiny video camera at the tip that is inserted into the rectum to allow the doctor to view the inside of the entire colon. The doctor may also biopsy the tissue and remove polyps during a colonoscopy.
- **Barium enema** - Chalky white liquid called barium is released into the colon (through the rectum) and then an X-ray is performed.
- **Digital rectal exam**

Diagnostic tests

If the screening tests or symptoms indicate the possibility of colorectal cancer, patients will undergo a diagnostic workup. These will help determine if colorectal cancer is present and the stage of the disease. Tests may include:

- **Medical history**
- **Physical exam**
- **Blood tests**
- **Biopsy** - abnormal tissue is removed and examined during a screening test to check for cancer cells.
- **Imaging Tests**
- **Ultrasound**
- **Computed tomography (CT)**
- **Magnetic resonance imaging (MRI)**
- **Chest X-ray** (to see if the cancer has spread to the lungs)

Treatments

Choice of treatment(s) depends on the location of the tumor (colon or rectum) and the stage of the disease. Common types of treatments include:

- **Surgery** - This is the most common treatment. It is used for removal of polyps and tumors and to check for the spread of the disease. Common types include laparoscopy and open surgery. After removal of part of the colon or rectum, the healthy parts are usually reconnected. When reconnection is not possible, a colostomy may be performed.
- **Chemotherapy** - Drug therapy that prevents the spread of cancer cells.
- **Radiation Therapy** - Also known as Radiotherapy, uses high energy-rays to kill cancer cells.
- **Biological Therapy** - Patients receive a monoclonal antibody through a vein which binds to colorectal cancer cells, interfering with their cell growth and spread in the body.

The Stages of Cancer

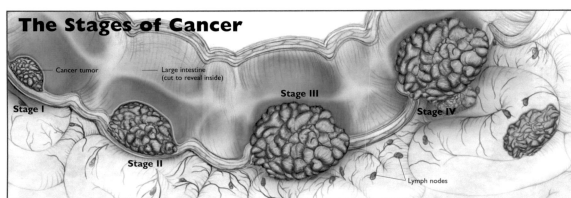

The earlier cancer is found and treated, the better the chances of getting well. The diagnosis of cancer is made by a microscopic test (biopsy) of a piece of tissue. Medical imaging techniques are used to measure how much the cancer has spread (grown) – this is known as staging.
The doctors often decide on the treatment based on the stage of cancer.

Doctors identify the stages of cancer as follows:

Stage I: The cancer has grown into the inner wall of the colon or rectum. The tumor has not yet reached the outer wall of the colon or extended outside the colon. Dukes' A is another name for Stage I colorectal cancer.

Stage II: The tumor extends more deeply into or through the wall of the colon or rectum. It may have invaded nearby tissue, but cancer cells have not yet spread to the lymph nodes. Dukes' B is another name for Stage II colorectal cancer.

Stage III: The cancer has spread to nearby lymph nodes, but not to other parts of the body. Dukes' C is another name for Stage III colorectal cancer.

Stage IV: The cancer has spread to other parts of the body, such as the liver or lungs. Dukes' D is another name for Stage IV colorectal cancer.

Cancer tumor

Large intestine (cut to reveal inside)

Stage I

Stage II

Stage III

Stage IV

Lymph nodes

Understanding the Common Cold

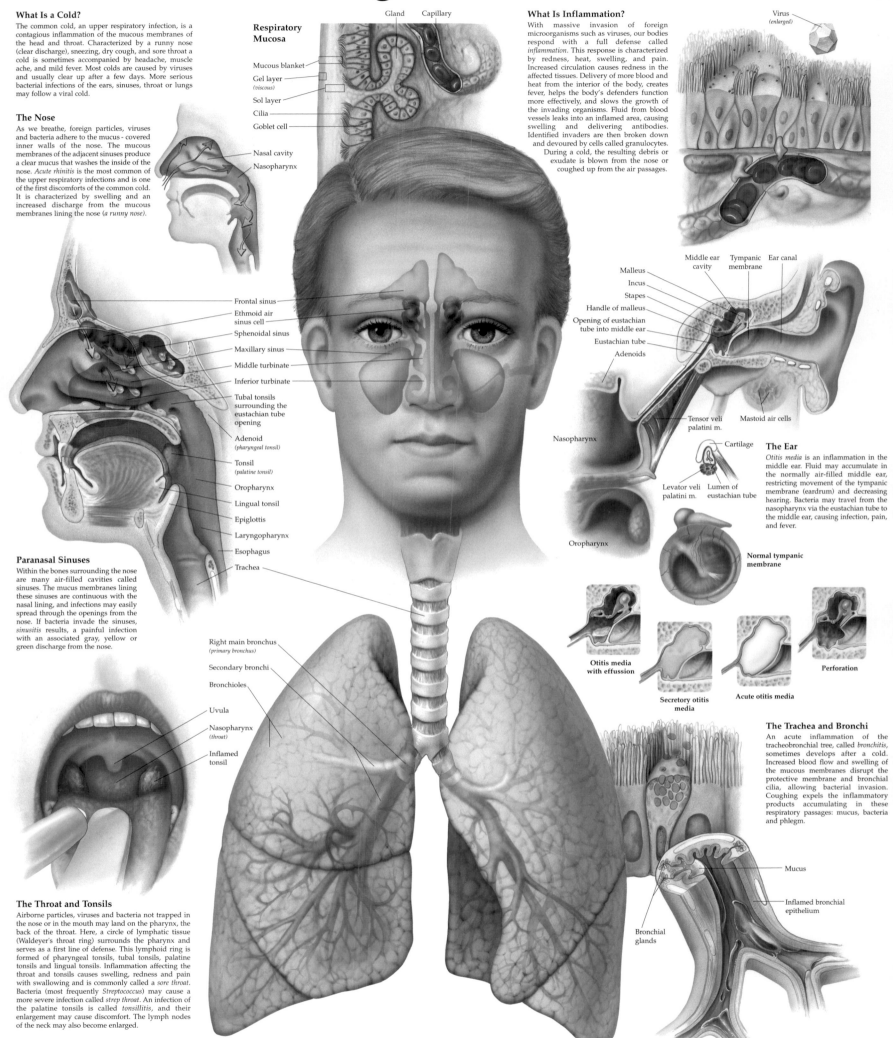

What Is a Cold?

The common cold, an upper respiratory infection, is a contagious inflammation of the mucous membranes of the head and throat. Characterized by a runny nose (clear discharge), sneezing, dry cough, and sore throat a cold is sometimes accompanied by headache, muscle ache, and mild fever. Most colds are caused by viruses and usually clear up after a few days. More serious bacterial infections of the ears, sinuses, throat or lungs may follow a viral cold.

The Nose

As we breathe, foreign particles, viruses and bacteria adhere to the mucus - covered inner walls of the nose. The mucous membranes of the adjacent sinuses produce a clear mucus that washes the inside of the nose. *Acute rhinitis* is the most common of the upper respiratory infections and is one of the first discomforts of the common cold. It is characterized by swelling and an increased discharge from the mucous membranes lining the nose (*a runny nose*).

Paranasal Sinuses

Within the bones surrounding the nose are many air-filled cavities called sinuses. The mucus membranes lining these sinuses are continuous with the nasal lining, and infections may easily spread through the openings from the nose. If bacteria invade the sinuses, *sinusitis* results, a painful infection with an associated gray, yellow or green discharge from the nose.

The Throat and Tonsils

Airborne particles, viruses and bacteria not trapped in the nose or in the mouth may land on the pharynx, the back of the throat. Here, a circle of lymphatic tissue (Waldeyer's throat ring) surrounds the pharynx and serves as a first line of defense. This lymphoid ring is formed of pharyngeal tonsils, tubal tonsils, palatine tonsils and lingual tonsils. Inflammation affecting the throat and tonsils causes swelling, redness and pain with swallowing and is commonly called a *sore throat*. Bacteria (most frequently *Streptococcus*) may cause a more severe infection called *strep throat*. An infection of the palatine tonsils is called *tonsillitis*, and their enlargement may cause discomfort. The lymph nodes of the neck may also become enlarged.

Respiratory Mucosa

- Gland
- Capillary
- Mucous blanket
- Gel layer (viscous)
- Sol layer
- Cilia
- Goblet cell

- Nasal cavity
- Nasopharynx

Labels (center figure):
- Frontal sinus
- Ethmoid air sinus cell
- Sphenoidal sinus
- Maxillary sinus
- Middle turbinate
- Inferior turbinate
- Tubal tonsils surrounding the eustachian tube opening
- Adenoid (pharyngeal tonsil)
- Tonsil (palatine tonsil)
- Oropharynx
- Lingual tonsil
- Epiglottis
- Laryngopharynx
- Esophagus
- Trachea

- Right main bronchus (primary bronchus)
- Secondary bronchi
- Bronchioles
- Uvula
- Nasopharynx (throat)
- Inflamed tonsil

What Is Inflammation?

With massive invasion of foreign microorganisms such as viruses, our bodies respond with a full defense called *inflammation*. This response is characterized by redness, heat, swelling, and pain. Increased circulation causes redness in the affected tissues. Delivery of more blood and heat from the interior of the body, creates fever, helps the body's defenders function more effectively, and slows the growth of the invading organisms. Fluid from blood vessels leaks into an inflamed area, causing swelling and delivering antibodies. Identified invaders are then broken down and devoured by cells called granulocytes. During a cold, the resulting debris or exudate is blown from the nose or coughed up from the air passages.

- Virus (enlarged)

The Ear

Otitis media is an inflammation in the middle ear. Fluid may accumulate in the normally air-filled middle ear, restricting movement of the tympanic membrane (eardrum) and decreasing hearing. Bacteria may travel from the nasopharynx via the eustachian tube to the middle ear, causing infection, pain, and fever.

Ear labels:
- Middle ear cavity
- Tympanic membrane
- Ear canal
- Malleus
- Incus
- Stapes
- Handle of malleus
- Opening of eustachian tube into middle ear
- Eustachian tube
- Adenoids
- Tensor veli palatini m.
- Mastoid air cells
- Nasopharynx
- Cartilage
- Levator veli palatini m.
- Lumen of eustachian tube
- Oropharynx
- Normal tympanic membrane

- Otitis media with effussion
- Secretory otitis media
- Acute otitis media
- Perforation

The Trachea and Bronchi

An acute inflammation of the tracheobronchial tree, called *bronchitis*, sometimes develops after a cold. Increased blood flow and swelling of the mucous membranes disrupt the protective membrane and bronchial cilia, allowing bacterial invasion. Coughing expels the inflammatory products accumulating in these respiratory passages: mucus, bacteria and phlegm.

- Mucus
- Inflamed bronchial epithelium
- Bronchial glands

Understanding Diabetes

What Is Diabetes?

Diabetes mellitus is the name for a group of chronic diseases that affect the way the body uses food to make the energy necessary for life. Diabetes is a disruption of carbohydrate (sugar and starch) metabolism, but it also affects fat and protein metabolism. This leads to hyperglycemia (increased blood glucose). High blood glucose for an extended period of time can result in damage to various parts of the body. There are two main forms of diabetes, Type 1 (insulin-dependent or juvenile) and Type 2 (non-insulin-dependent or adult-onset). Some secondary forms also exist, caused by conditions such as pancreatic disease, pregnancy (gestational diabetes mellitus), hormonal or genetic problems, and certain drugs.

Brain

Lung

Heart

Liver

Stomach

Pancreas

Kidney

Large intestine

Small intestine

Type 1 Diabetes

Type 1 diabetes is a disease in which the pancreas produces little or no insulin. Insulin is needed to transport glucose into the cells for use as energy and storage as glycogen (sugar). It also stimulates protein synthesis and free fatty acid storage in the fat deposits. When a person lacks sufficient insulin, body tissues have less access to essential nutrients for fuel and storage. Type 1 diabetes usually develops before age 30, although it may strike at any age.

Type 2 Diabetes

In Type 2 diabetes, the pancreas produces some insulin, but it is either too little or is not effective. Also, insulin receptors that control the transport of glucose into cells may not work properly (insulin resistance) or are reduced in number. The more common form of diabetes, Type 2 typically develops in adults over age 40, but it can appear earlier. Type 2 diabetes may also develop as a consequence of obesity.

Potential Complications of Diabetes:

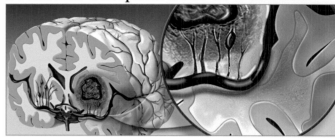

Stroke: Causing loss of neurologic function, leading to numbness, weakness, difficulty with speech, coordination, or walking.

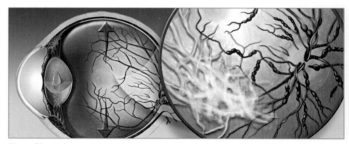

Eye disease: Causing blind spots or blindness.

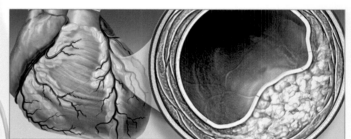

Heart disease: Causing heart attacks and congestive heart failure.

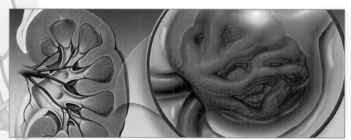

Kidney disease: Causing kidney failure.

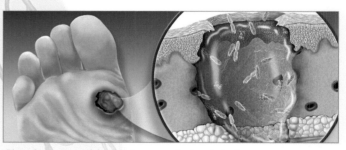

Circulatory problems: Causing sores that do not heal well. In extreme situations, gangrene can develop and can lead to amputations.

What Are the Symptoms of Diabetes?

Patients with **Type 1 diabetes** usually report rapidly developing symptoms. With **Type 2 diabetes**, symptoms usually develop gradually and may not appear until many years after the onset of the disease.

Some of the symptoms for Type 1 or Type 2 diabetes are included in the following list.

- Sudden weight loss
- Frequent urination
- Extreme hunger
- Excessive thirst
- Blurred vision
- Dry, itchy skin

- More infections than usual
- Numbness in feet, hands
- Slow-healing cuts or sores
- Fatigue or tiredness
- No symptoms

What Are the Long-Term Health Problems?

High blood glucose levels caused by diabetes may damage small and large blood vessels and nerves. Diabetes may also lower the body's ability to fight infection. Because of these changes, people with diabetes are more likely to have serious eye problems, kidney disease, heart attacks, strokes, high blood pressure, circulatory problems, numbness of the feet, sexual problems, and infections. Patients with diabetes should be checked regularly for signs of these complications, many of which can be reduced or delayed with good blood glucose control and regular medical care.

Cardiovascular Disease

NORMAL HEART ANATOMY

Cross Section

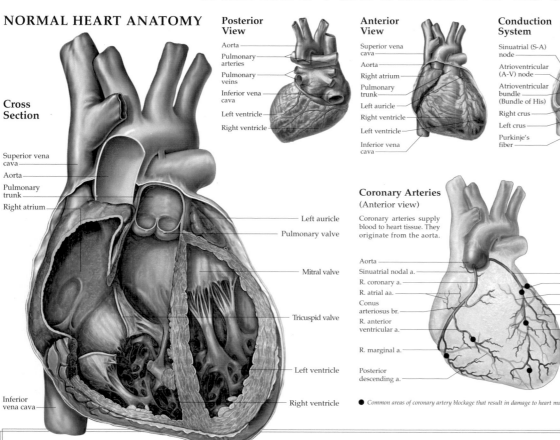

- Superior vena cava
- Aorta
- Pulmonary trunk
- Right atrium
- Left auricle
- Pulmonary valve
- Mitral valve
- Tricuspid valve
- Left ventricle
- Inferior vena cava
- Right ventricle

Posterior View

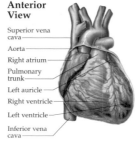

- Aorta
- Pulmonary arteries
- Pulmonary veins
- Inferior vena cava
- Left ventricle
- Right ventricle

Anterior View

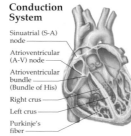

- Superior vena cava
- Aorta
- Right atrium
- Pulmonary trunk
- Left auricle
- Right ventricle
- Left ventricle
- Inferior vena cava

Conduction System

- Sinuatrial (S-A) node
- Atrioventricular (A-V) node
- Atrioventricular bundle (Bundle of His)
- Right crus
- Left crus
- Purkinje's fiber

Coronary Arteries (Anterior view)

Coronary arteries supply blood to heart tissue. They originate from the aorta.

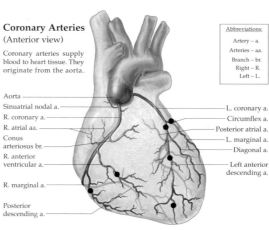

- Aorta
- Sinuatrial nodal a.
- R. coronary a.
- R. atrial aa.
- Conus arteriosus br.
- R. anterior ventricular a.
- R. marginal a.
- Posterior descending a.
- L. coronary a.
- Circumflex a.
- Posterior atrial a.
- L. marginal a.
- Diagonal a.
- Left anterior descending a.

Abbreviations:
- Artery – a.
- Arteries – aa.
- Branch – br.
- Right – R.
- Left – L.

● *Common areas of coronary artery blockage that result in damage to heart muscle.*

Electrocardiogram (ECG)

Repeating electrical impulses travel through the heart, controlling the rhythmic contraction and dilation of the heart muscle. The impulse is displayed in a waveform with three distinct waves: P, QRS, and T.

The Cardiac Cycle

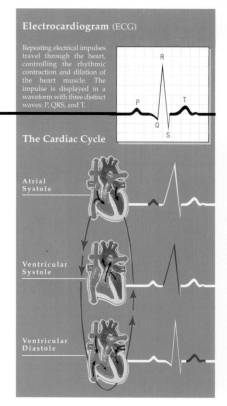

- Atrial Systole
- Ventricular Systole
- Ventricular Diastole

CARDIOVASCULAR DISEASE

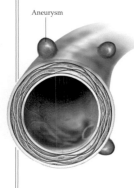

- Aneurysm
- Inflammation of blood vessel

Polyarteritis Nodosa (PAN)

Polyarteritis nodosa (PAN) is a disease of inflammation of the small and medium-sized blood vessels, which can involve multiple organs of the body. The organs most commonly involved are the kidneys, heart, liver, and gastrointestinal tract. Less commonly involved are the muscles, brain, spinal cord, peripheral nerves, and skin. The inflammation can cause beadlike aneurysms of the involved blood vessels, which cause decreased blood flow to the affected organs.

Kawasaki's Disease

Also known as mucocutaneous lymph node syndrome, Kawasaki's disease is a multi-organ illness affecting children. It generally starts with high fever, followed by the development of redness and swelling of the hands, feet, eyes, lips, and tongue; swollen lymph glands; and sores in the mouth. Acute complications involving the heart include inflammation of the heart muscle and accumulation of fluid around the heart. Fatal heart attacks occur due to inflammation of the blood vessels (coronary arteries) of the heart, causing blood clots to form and block the arteries. Chronic complications include aneurysms of the coronary arteries that can rupture in adulthood.

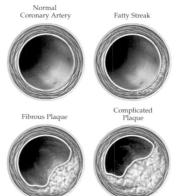

- Normal Coronary Artery
- Fatty Streak
- Fibrous Plaque
- Complicated Plaque

Coronary Artery Disease

If excessive amounts of fat are circulating in the blood, the arteries can accumulate fatty deposits called plaques. This buildup, called atherosclerosis, causes the vessels to narrow or become obstructed. Coronary artery disease results as atherosclerotic plaque fills the lumens of the coronary arteries and obstructs blood flow to the heart. This results in diminished supply of oxygen and nutrients to the heart tissue.

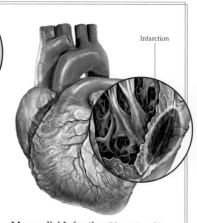

- Blocked artery

Angina

The coronary arteries supplying the heart can become narrowed over time, due to age, hereditary factors, chronic smoking, high cholesterol, high blood pressure, or diabetes. The narrowed blood vessels limit the amount of blood flow to the heart, especially with strenuous activity. When the heart muscle is not getting enough blood, pain or discomfort in the chest, commonly called angina, results.

- Infarction

Myocardial Infarction (Heart Attack)

Myocardial infarction occurs when a coronary artery narrowed by atherosclerosis becomes completely blocked. This is usually the result of a blood clot that forms where the artery is narrowed. The blocked artery prevents the heart from receiving oxygen, and part or all of the heart muscle is either damaged (infarction) or dies. The damaged part of the heart loses its ability to contract and pump blood to and from the heart.

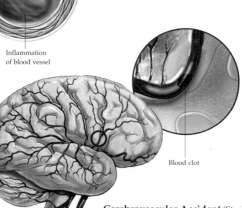

- Blood clot

Cerebrovascular Accident (Stroke)

A cerebrovascular accident (CVA), also known as a stroke, is a sudden impairment of cerebral circulation in one or more blood vessels. This interrupts or diminishes oxygen supply to the brain, often causing the brain tissues to become damaged or die.

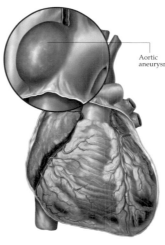

- Aortic aneurysm

Aortic Aneurysm

The aorta is the largest blood vessel in the body. It comes out of the top of the heart and brings blood to the rest of the body. Atherosclerosis can cause the wall of the aorta to weaken and balloon out (aneurysm). The aortic aneurysm may suddenly rupture or tear, often leading to death.

- Thickened heart muscle

Left Ventricular Hypertrophy (LVH)

LVH is when the muscle of the heart's left ventricle becomes thickened and enlarged. The heart then becomes less efficient at circulating blood throughout the body. The resulting condition is called congestive heart failure. This may cause the lungs to fill up with fluid, resulting in difficulty breathing, fluid retention and swollen legs, and decreased blood flow to various parts of the body.

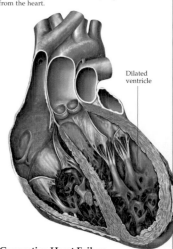

- Dilated ventricle

Congestive Heart Failure

Congestive heart failure is a common debilitating condition defined by the heart's mechanical inability to pump blood effectively. The result is a decrease in blood circulation, which forces blood to back up and oxygen supply to decrease in muscle and lung tissues. Excess accumulation of fluids in tissues throughout the body causes swelling (edema), which impairs the function of affected organs.

Chronic Obstructive Pulmonary Disease (COPD)

Chronic Obstructive Pulmonary Disease (COPD)

Chronic obstructive pulmonary disease (COPD) is a term used to describe prolonged irreversible airflow obstruction that is mainly associated with emphysema and chronic bronchitis.

The most common chronic lung disease, COPD is a leading global health problem causing significant worldwide disability. COPD is the 4th leading cause of death and unfortunately its prevalence continues to rise. Early on, it does not always produce symptoms and causes only minimal disability in many patients. However, COPD tends to worsen with time.

Emphysema

In normal, healthy breathing, air moves in and out of the lungs to meet metabolic needs. Any change in airway size compromises the lungs' ability to circulate sufficient air.

In a patient with emphysema, recurrent pulmonary inflammation damages and eventually destroys the alveolar walls, causing them to break down and merge, creating large air spaces. This breakdown leaves the alveoli unable to recoil normally after expanding and results in bronchiolar collapse on exhalation. This traps air within the lungs, causing breathlessness.

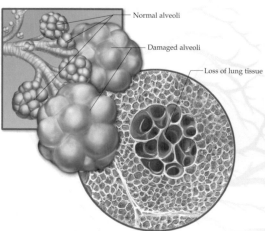

Normal alveoli
Damaged alveoli
Loss of lung tissue

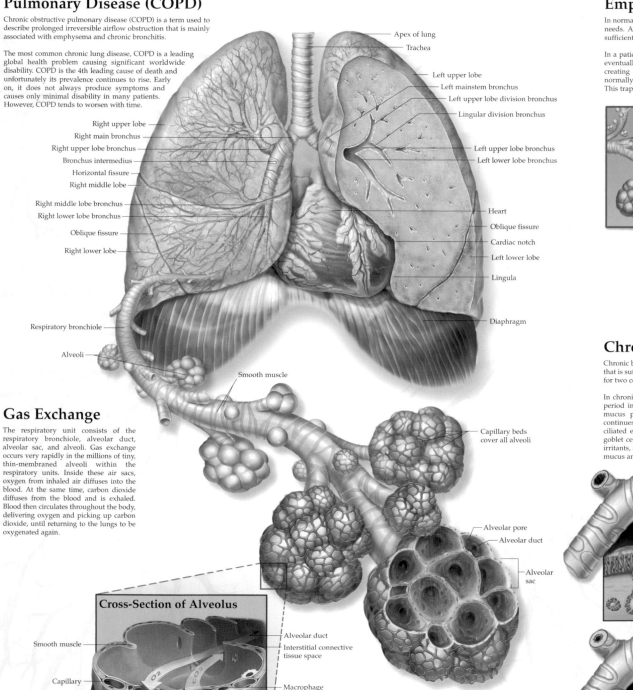

Apex of lung
Trachea
Left upper lobe
Left mainstem bronchus
Left upper lobe division bronchus
Lingular division bronchus
Left upper lobe bronchus
Left lower lobe bronchus
Right upper lobe
Right main bronchus
Right upper lobe bronchus
Bronchus intermedius
Horizontal fissure
Right middle lobe
Right middle lobe bronchus
Right lower lobe bronchus
Oblique fissure
Right lower lobe
Heart
Oblique fissure
Cardiac notch
Left lower lobe
Lingula
Diaphragm
Respiratory bronchiole
Alveoli
Smooth muscle
Capillary beds cover all alveoli
Alveolar pore
Alveolar duct
Alveolar sac

Gas Exchange

The respiratory unit consists of the respiratory bronchiole, alveolar duct, alveolar sac, and alveoli. Gas exchange occurs very rapidly in the millions of tiny, thin-membraned alveoli within the respiratory units. Inside these air sacs, oxygen from inhaled air diffuses into the blood. At the same time, carbon dioxide diffuses from the blood and is exhaled. Blood then circulates throughout the body, delivering oxygen and picking up carbon dioxide, until returning to the lungs to be oxygenated again.

Cross-Section of Alveolus

Smooth muscle
Capillary
Elastic fibers
Fibroblast
Alveolar cell:
Type I pneumocyte
Type II pneumocyte
Alveolar duct
Interstitial connective tissue space
Macrophage
Basal lamina
Collagen fibril

Chronic Bronchitis

Chronic bronchitis is marked by excessive production of tracheobronchial mucus that is sufficient to cause a cough on most days for at least three months each year for two consecutive years.

In chronic bronchitis, irritants such as cigarette smoke inhaled for a prolonged period inflame the tracheobronchial tree. The inflammation leads to increased mucus production and a narrowed or blocked airway. As inflammation continues, the mucus-producing goblet cells undergo hypertrophy, as do the ciliated epithelial cells that line the respiratory tract. Hypersecretion from the goblet cells blocks the free movement of the cilia, which normally sweep dust, irritants, and mucus from the airways. As a result, the airway stays blocked, and mucus and debris accumulate in the respiratory tract.

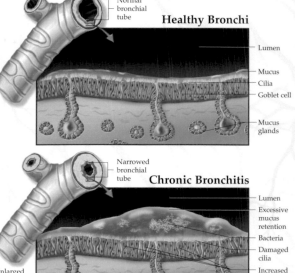

Normal bronchial tube
Healthy Bronchi
Lumen
Mucus
Cilia
Goblet cell
Mucus glands

Narrowed bronchial tube
Chronic Bronchitis
Lumen
Excessive mucus retention
Bacteria
Damaged cilia
Enlarged mucous glands
Increased number of goblet cells

Causes

Predisposing factors to COPD include:
- cigarette smoking
- recurrent or chronic respiratory infections
- air pollution
- allergies

Smoking is by far the most important of these factors. Smoking increases mucus production and impairs its removal from the airways, impedes the function of airway cells that digest disease-causing organisms, causes airway inflammation, destroys air sacs in the lungs, and leads to abnormal fibrous tissue growth in the bronchial tree.

Early inflammatory changes may reverse themselves if the person stops smoking before lung damage is extensive. Hereditary factors (such as deficiency of alpha-1 antitrypsin) may also predispose a person to the development of COPD.

Symptoms

The typical COPD patient is a long-term smoker who has no symptoms until middle age, when his or her ability to exercise or do strenuous work starts to decline and a productive cough begins.

Subtle at first, these problems worsen as the patient ages and the disease progresses. Eventually, they cause difficulty breathing even on minimal exertion, frequent respiratory infections, oxygen deficiency in the blood, and abnormalities in pulmonary function.

When advanced, chronic bronchitis and emphysema may cause chest deformities, overwhelming disability, heart enlargement, severe respiratory failure, and death.

Diagnosis

Chest X-rays
Help to rule out pneumonia and lung cancer. They also show heart size. If the patient has emphysema, X-rays can pinpoint areas of damaged lung tissue.

Pulmonary Function Tests
Measure lung capacity and airway obstruction.

Arterial Blood Gas Analysis
Measures the amount of oxygen and carbon dioxide in the blood.

Electrocardiography
Measures the electric activity of the heart.

Sputum Analysis
Detects respiratory infection.

Treatment

Since the majority of cases of COPD are smoking-related, the patient should **avoid smoking**.

The main goal of treatment is to relieve symptoms and prevent complications. **Bronchodilators** can help alleviate bronchospasm and enhance mucociliary clearance of secretions. **Effective coughing, postural drainage, and chest physiotherapy** can help mobilize secretions.

In patients who require it, administration of low concentrations of **oxygen** helps relieve symptoms and prolongs life.

Antibiotics allow treatment of respiratory infections. **Pneumococcal vaccination and annual influenza vaccinations** are important in preventing complications.

Pulmonary rehabilitation improves quality of life, strength, and sense of well-being.

©2008 Wolters Kluwer | Lippincott Williams & Wilkins | Published by Anatomical Chart Company, Skokie, IL
Health

Understanding Depression

What Is Depression?

Clinical depression is a serious medical condition that affects thoughts, mood, feelings, behavior, and physical health. Clinical depression is persistent and can interfere significantly with an individual's ability to function. Depression is one of the most common mental health disorders and is the leading cause of disability in the U.S. and worldwide. In the U.S., it affects about one in five people at some time in life. Twice as many women as men experience depression. There are three main types of depressive disorders: major depressive disorder, dysthymic disorder, and bipolar disorder.

Neuron Structure

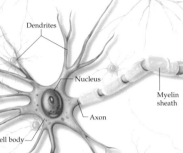

Dendrites
Nucleus
Axon
Cell body
Myelin sheath
Node of Ranvier

The Role of Neurotransmitters

Neurotransmitters are chemical messengers that carry messages between neurons (nerve cells) and affect behavior, mood, and thought. They are released into the synapses (gaps) between neurons to help messages travel from one cell to another. Two of the neurotransmitters that play a role in depression are **norepinephrine** and **serotonin**. Low levels of these neurotransmitters in areas of the brain that control mood and emotion may result in depression.

1 Nerve message
Synaptic vesicles
2 Release of neurotransmitter molecules (norepinephrine and serotonin)
Synaptic cleft
3 Neurotransmitters bind to receptor sites
4 Membrane channels open as result of binding of neurotransmitters
5 Nerve message is transmitted to adjoining neuron
Dendrite of receiving neuron

In depression, neurons don't produce enough neurotransmitters. As a result, membrane channels don't open, nerve messages are not communicated, and areas of the brain affecting emotion may not receive stimulation.

Closed membrane channels

Hypothalamic-Pituitary-Adrenal Axis

Evidence suggests that the hormonal system known as the **hypothalamic-pituitary-adrenal (HPA) axis**, which regulates the body's response to stress, is overactive in many people with depression. The hypothalamus increases production of **corticotropin releasing factor (CRF)** when a person's physical or psychological well-being is threatened. Elevated levels of CRF lead to an increase in hormone secretion by the pituitary and adrenal glands which prepares the body for defensive action. Research indicates that chronic overactivity of the HPA axis, as may occur following a traumatic experience, may contribute to the onset of depression.

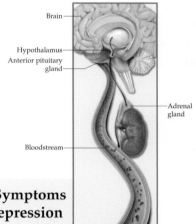

Brain
Hypothalamus
Anterior pituitary gland
Bloodstream
Adrenal gland

Areas of the Brain Affected by Depression

Several areas of the brain are involved in the emotional and physical changes seen in depression. While the brain of a depressed individual is generally underactive, certain areas display overactivity.

Thalamus
The thalamus is associated with changes in emotion and is known to stimulate the amygdala. This area displays increased levels of activity in depressed individuals.

Cingulate gyrus
In depression, there is increased activity in the cingulate gyrus. This area helps associate smells and sights with pleasant memories of past emotions. It also takes part in the emotional reaction to pain and the regulation of aggression.

Prefrontal cortex
Parts of the prefrontal cortex help regulate emotion. People who are depressed have decreased activity in this section of the brain.

Amygdala
The amygdala, which is responsible for negative feelings, displays overactivity in depressed people.

The Limbic System

The limbic system plays a complex and important role in the expression of instincts, drives, and emotions. It mediates the effects of moods on external behavior and influences internal changes in bodily functions associated with depression.

Fornix
Thalamus
Hippocampus
Parahippocampal gyrus
Mamillary body
Amygdala

Three Main Types of Depression

Major Depression

A diagnosis of major depression is made if a person has five or more symptoms of depression and has impairment in functioning nearly every day during a two-week period.

Dysthymic Disorder (Dysthymia)

A chronic but less severe form of depression, dysthymia, is diagnosed when a person's depressed mood persists for at least two years and is accompanied by two other symptoms of depression. Signs and symptoms usually aren't disabling, and periods of dysthymia can alternate with short periods of feeling normal. Dysthymia puts a person at increased risk for developing major depression.

Bipolar Disorder (Manic-Depressive Illness)

Bipolar disorder is characterized by distinct and recurrent episodes of elevated mood (mania), often alternating with episodes of depression. Symptoms of mania include overly inflated self-esteem, decreased need for sleep, increased talkativeness, racing thoughts, distractibility, excessive risk taking, extreme irritability, and poor judgment.

Signs and Symptoms of Major Depression

Changes that include five or more of the following symptoms for more than two weeks at any one time, indicate depression and should be reported to a healthcare provider.

- Loss of interest or enjoyment in normal daily activities
- Persistent sad, anxious, or hopeless mood
- Irritability or agitation
- Feelings of guilt, fear, or worthlessness
- Significant weight loss or gain
- Significant changes in appetite
- Impaired thinking or concentration
- Fatigue
- Insomnia or excessive sleeping
- Thoughts of death or suicide
- Unexplained crying spells
- Difficulty making decisions
- Decreased sex drive

Risk Factors

There are several factors that can contribute to the development of depression.

- **Heredity**–Research has identified genes that may be involved in bipolar disorder. Not everyone with a family history of depression develops the disorder.
- **Stress**–Traumatic experiences, such as the loss of a loved one, can trigger depression.
- **Physical Disorders**–Chronic illnesses, such as heart disease, hypothyroidism, stroke, neurological disorders, and some infections can put a person at higher risk for developing depression.
- **Hormonal Changes**–Women may be vulnerable to depression due to changing hormone levels, as in postpartum depression.
- **Alcohol, Nicotine, and Drug Abuse**–These substances may contribute to depression.
- **Diet**–Symptoms of depression may be caused by deficiencies in folic acid and vitamin B-12.

Suicide

Depression is a serious illness that, if left untreated, can result in more frequent and severe episodes over time. It can lead to a downward spiral of disability, dependency, and suicide.

Certain warning signs may indicate serious depression and any threat of suicide should be taken seriously. If you see any of the following danger signs contact a doctor, mental health clinic, or suicide hotline immediately.

- Pacing, agitated behavior, frequent mood changes
- Actions or threats of physical harm or violence
- Threats or talk of death or suicide
- Withdrawal from activities and relationships
- Giving away prized possessions or saying goodbye to friends
- A sudden brightening of mood after a period of severe depression
- Unusually risky behavior

Treatment

Depression can almost always be treated effectively. The first step is a physical examination by a physician. Certain medications and medical conditions can cause the same symptoms as depression and must be ruled out before a diagnosis of depression is made. If depression is diagnosed, treatment can include one or more of the following:

Antidepressants

These medications work by influencing the functioning of targeted chemicals in the brain. Types of antidepressants include:

- **Selective serotonin reuptake inhibitors (SSRIs)**- Increase availability of serotonin.
- **Tricyclics (TCAs)**-Increase the levels of serotonin and norepinephrine.
- **Monoamine oxidase inhibitors (MAOIs)**- Prevent the breakdown of excitatory neurotransmitters (monoamines).

Mood Stabilizers

Patients with bipolar disorder are at risk of switching into hypomania (mild to moderate mania) to severe mania when taking antidepressant medication. For this reason, mood stabilizers are usually prescribed alone or in combination with antidepressants for the treatment of bipolar disorder.

Psychotherapy

- **Cognitive-behavioral therapy (CBT)**-Targeted at changing negative, self-defeating thought patterns and behaviors.
- **Interpersonal therapy (IPT) and group psychotherapy**-Focus on interpersonal relationships and improving communication skills and social support.
- **Psychodynamic therapy**-Focuses on resolving the patient's conflicted feelings and making characterological changes.

Alternative Therapies

- **Herbal therapy**-Herbal products may have a beneficial effect in mild cases of depression. Patients should talk with their doctor before taking any herbal or dietary supplement. Studies are being done to determine the effectiveness of these remedies.
- **Exercise**- Exercise may be useful in mild cases of depression. Increased physical activity helps by boosting serotonin levels in the body.

©2008 Wolters Kluwer | Lippincott Williams & Wilkins | Published by Anatomical Chart Company, Skokie, IL
Health

Diseases of the Digestive System

45

Hiatal hernia

Achalasia

Squamous carcinoma of esophagus

Stenosing web of esophagus

Barrett's esophagus

Adenocarcinoma of esophagus

Esophageal varices

Postnecrotic cirrhosis

Cirrhosis

Fatty liver

Viral hepatitis

Gastric ulcer

Bacterial hepatitis

Gallstones in: Cystic duct Gall bladder

Adenocarcinoma of stomach

Adenocarcinoma of pancreas

Normal liver

Duodenal ulcer

Gallstones in common bile duct

Acute and chronic gastritis

Acute pancreatitis

Colonic polyps

Circumferencial carcinoma of transverse colon

Adenocarcinoma of colon

Inflammatory bowel disease: Ulcerative colitis Crohn's Disease (Granulomatous Colitis)

Adenocarcinoma of jejunum

Intussuception caused by polyp

Fecalith obstructing lumen causing appendicitis

Diverticulosis of colon

Indirect inquinal hernia

Ulcerative colitis

Adenocarcinoma of rectosigmoid region

Internal hemorrhoids

External hemorrhoids

©2008 Wolters Kluwer | Lippincott Williams & Wilkins | Published by Anatomical Chart Company, Skokie, IL

Gastroesophageal Disorders and Digestive Anatomy

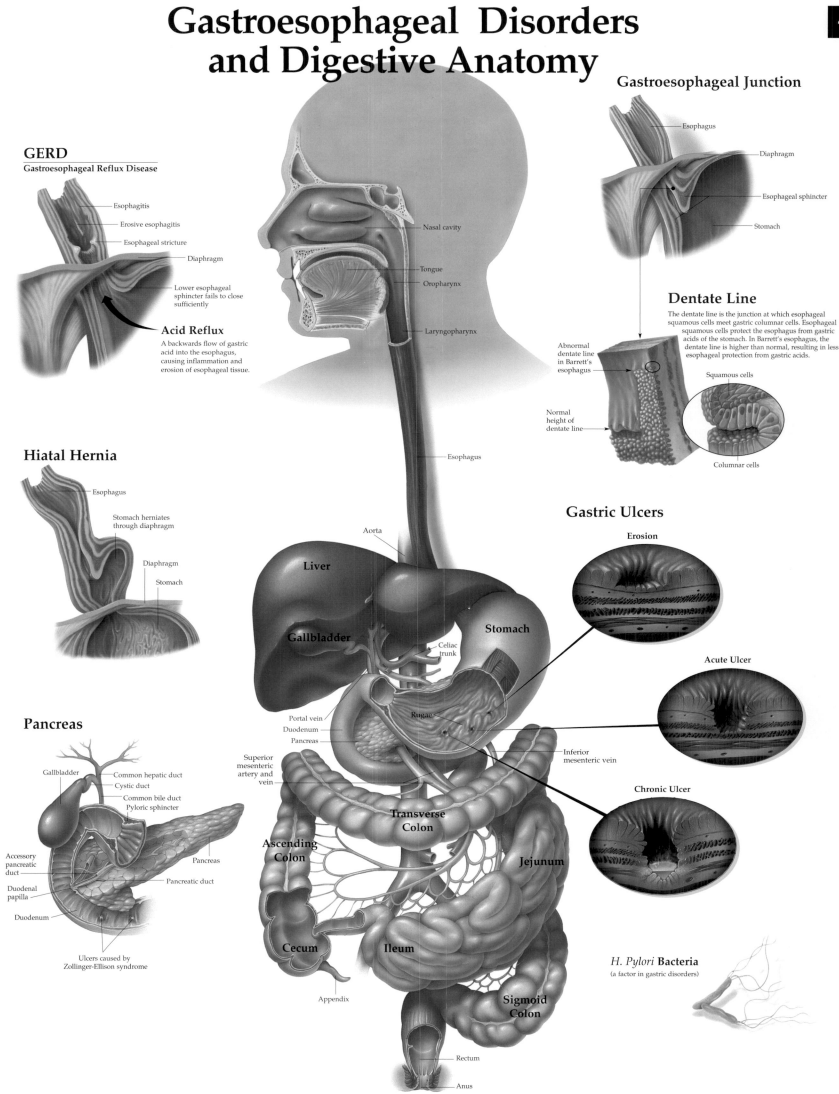

46

GERD
Gastroesophageal Reflux Disease

- Esophagitis
- Erosive esophagitis
- Esophageal stricture
- Diaphragm
- Lower esophageal sphincter fails to close sufficiently

Acid Reflux

A backwards flow of gastric acid into the esophagus, causing inflammation and erosion of esophageal tissue.

Hiatal Hernia

- Esophagus
- Stomach herniates through diaphragm
- Diaphragm
- Stomach

Pancreas

- Gallbladder
- Common hepatic duct
- Cystic duct
- Common bile duct
- Pyloric sphincter
- Pancreas
- Accessory pancreatic duct
- Pancreatic duct
- Duodenal papilla
- Duodenum
- Ulcers caused by Zollinger-Ellison syndrome

Central figure labels

- Nasal cavity
- Tongue
- Oropharynx
- Laryngopharynx
- Esophagus
- Aorta
- Liver
- Gallbladder
- Celiac trunk
- Stomach
- Portal vein
- Duodenum
- Pancreas
- Rugae
- Superior mesenteric artery and vein
- Inferior mesenteric vein
- Transverse Colon
- Ascending Colon
- Jejunum
- Cecum
- Ileum
- Appendix
- Sigmoid Colon
- Rectum
- Anus

Gastroesophageal Junction

- Esophagus
- Diaphragm
- Esophageal sphincter
- Stomach

Dentate Line

The dentate line is the junction at which esophageal squamous cells meet gastric columnar cells. Esophageal squamous cells protect the esophagus from gastric acids of the stomach. In Barrett's esophagus, the dentate line is higher than normal, resulting in less esophageal protection from gastric acids.

- Abnormal dentate line in Barrett's esophagus
- Squamous cells
- Normal height of dentate line
- Columnar cells

Gastric Ulcers

Erosion

Acute Ulcer

Chronic Ulcer

H. Pylori **Bacteria**
(a factor in gastric disorders)

Human Spine Disorders

47

The Spinal Column (Lateral View)

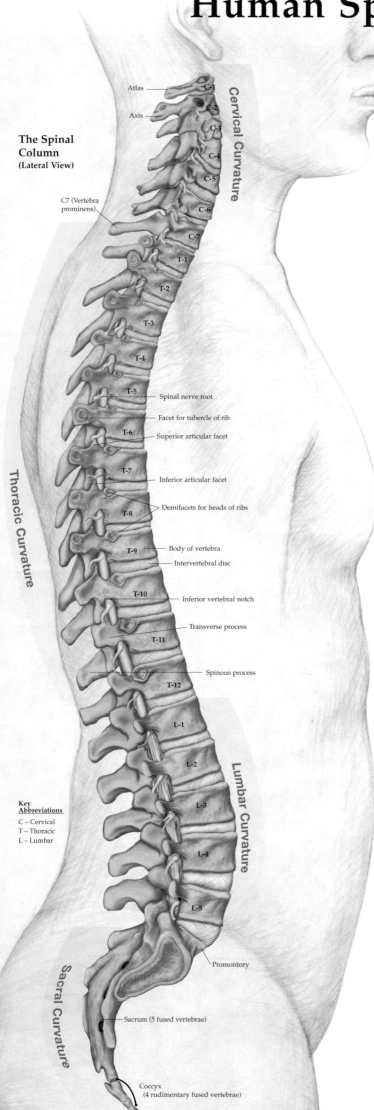

Atlas — C-1
Axis — C-2
C-3
C-4
C-5
C7 (Vertebra prominens)
C-6
C-7
Cervical Curvature
T-1
T-2
T-3
T-4
T-5 — Spinal nerve root
— Facet for tubercle of rib
T-6 — Superior articular facet
T-7 — Inferior articular facet
T-8 — Demifacets for heads of ribs
T-9 — Body of vertebra
— Intervertebral disc
T-10 — Inferior vertebral notch
— Transverse process
T-11
T-12 — Spinous process
Thoracic Curvature
L-1
L-2
L-3
L-4
L-5
Lumbar Curvature
Promontory
Sacrum (5 fused vertebrae)
Sacral Curvature
Coccyx (4 rudimentary fused vertebrae)

Key Abbreviations
C – Cervical
T – Thoracic
L – Lumbar

Anatomy

A Typical Cervical Vertebra (Superior View)

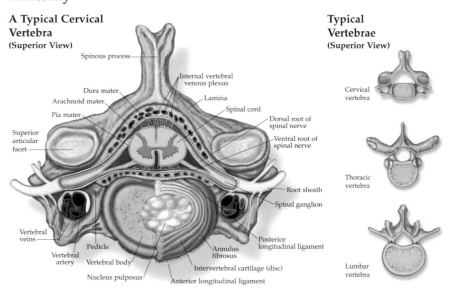

Spinous process
Internal vertebral venous plexus
Dura mater
Arachnoid mater
Pia mater
Lamina
Spinal cord
Dorsal root of spinal nerve
Superior articular facet
Ventral root of spinal nerve
Root sheath
Spinal ganglion
Vertebral veins
Posterior longitudinal ligament
Vertebral artery
Pedicle
Vertebral body
Annulus fibrosus
Nucleus pulposus
Intervertebral cartilage (disc)
Anterior longitudinal ligament

Typical Vertebrae (Superior View)

Cervical vertebra
Thoracic vertebra
Lumbar vertebra

Structural Features of an Intervertebral Disc (Schematic)

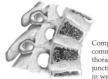

Nucleus pulposus
Annulus fibrosus

Note alternating obliquity of collagen fibrils.

The nucleus pulposus is the central gelatinous cushioning part of the intervertebral disc enclosed in several layers of cartilaginous laminae. The nucleus pulposus becomes dehydrated with age.

Function of Intervertebral Discs

Normal   Weight

Body
Disc
Annulus fibrosus
Nucleus pulposus

The disc, which contains nucleus pulposus, functions to protect the vertebrae from pressure.

Pathology

Osteoporosis

Osteoporosis develops when the body loses bone more quickly than it can make new bone. As a result, bones become less dense at the core and lose thickness at the surface. This increases the bones' susceptibility to fracture.

When osteoporosis involves the lumbar region, the vertebral bodies become markedly biconcave and the discs are ballooned.

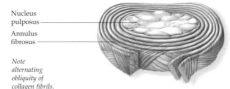

Compression fractures * commonly occur at the thoracolumbar vertebral junction, resulting in wedge-shaped vertebrae.

* Fractures of laminae, pedicles, or transverse processes of the vertebrae are common.

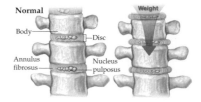

A. Hyperkyphosis
An excessive rounding of the thoracic vertebral column (humpback or hunchback).

B. Scoliosis
A curvature of the spine, often with twisting of the spinal column.

C. Hyperlordosis
A forward/anterior curvature of the cervical and lumbar (lower back) regions of the spine. In the lumbar region, it is also called "swayback."

Causes of Pain in the Back or Extremities

Shown below are other causes of pain that the examining physician should consider in making the diagnosis.

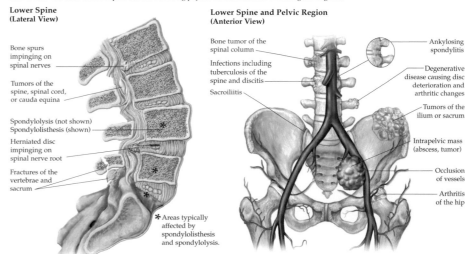

Lower Spine (Lateral View)

Bone spurs impinging on spinal nerves
Tumors of the spine, spinal cord, or cauda equina
Spondylolysis (not shown)
Spondylolisthesis (shown)
Herniated disc impinging on spinal nerve root
Fractures of the vertebrae and sacrum

* Areas typically affected by spondylolisthesis and spondylolysis.

Lower Spine and Pelvic Region (Anterior View)

Bone tumor of the spinal column
Infections including tuberculosis of the spine and discitis
Sacroiliitis
Ankylosing spondylitis
Degenerative disease causing disc deterioration and arthritic changes
Tumors of the ilium or sacrum
Intrapelvic mass (abscess, tumor)
Occlusion of vessels
Arthritis of the hip

©2008 Wolters Kluwer Health | Lippincott Williams & Wilkins | Published by Anatomical Chart Company, Skokie, IL

48

Hypertension

What Is Hypertension?

Hypertension or **high blood pressure** is a disorder marked by intermittent or consistent elevation of diastolic and/or systolic blood pressure. Generally, a sustained systolic pressure of 140 mmHg or more, or a diastolic pressure of 90 mmHg or more, qualifies as hypertension. The risk to the patient lies in the long-term damage that hypertension can cause to the brain, eyes, heart, blood vessels, and kidneys.

Normal Blood Pressure		
Systolic mmHg	=	120 mmHg
Diastolic mmHg		80 mmHg

High Blood Pressure		
Systolic mmHg	≥	140 mmHg
Diastolic mmHg		90 mmHg

What Is Blood Pressure (BP)?

As blood is pumped through the body, it creates pressure within the arteries. This pressure is referred to as blood pressure. A blood pressure reading indicates arterial pressure during the heart's contraction (systole) and dilation (diastole). Blood pressure measurement is an important tool to assess the functioning of the heart, kidneys, and blood vessels.

Types and Causes of Hypertension

Essential hypertension is the most common type of hypertension, yet its cause is unknown. Family medical history, race, stress, obesity, a diet high in sodium or saturated fat, use of tobacco and oral contraceptives, sedentary lifestyle, and aging have been studied to determine their role in the development of hypertension.

Secondary hypertension may result from renal vascular disease, renal parenchymal disease, pheochromocytoma, Cushing's syndrome, diabetes mellitus, dysfunction of the thyroid or pituitary gland, pregnancy, and some neurologic disorders.

What Are the Common Symptoms of Hypertension?

Hypertension generally does *not* cause any symptoms. It is often diagnosed when a patient visits the doctor for a routine check-up. Rarely, headaches can result from extremely high blood pressure. Other symptoms are generally related to the potential complications of chronic hypertension, such as sudden blurred or loss of vision; dizziness; numbness, tingling, or weakness of a part of the body; trouble with coordination; chest pain; shortness of breath; palpitations (irregular heartbeats); abdominal pain; swelling; and weight gain due to fluid retention.

Potential Complications of Hypertension

Brain

Cerebrovascular Accident (Stroke)

Hypertension is the major cause of stroke. Long-term high blood pressure can cause hardening and narrowing of the blood vessels in the brain. A blood clot can then form at the area of the narrowed blood vessel and stop blood flow to that part of the brain, resulting in damage to the brain tissue (stroke).

Under increasing blood pressure, a weakening of the artery wall may balloon out (aneurysm) and burst, causing hemorrhage (bleeding), brain damage, and even death.

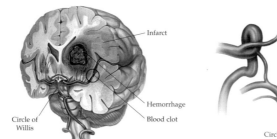

Infarct
Hemorrhage
Blood clot
Circle of Willis

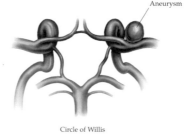

Aneurysm
Circle of Willis

Eye

Hypertensive Retinopathy

Long-term hypertension can cause hardening (arteriosclerosis) of the blood vessels in the inside part of the eye called the retina. Potential complications of hardening of blood vessels include severe narrowing of the vessels. As the disease progresses, flame-shaped hemorrhages (bleeding) and cotton-wool spots develop. Leaking from the retinal vessels can cause hard exudates to form. Because of increased pressure, the optic disk may become swollen. These complications can lead to blindness.

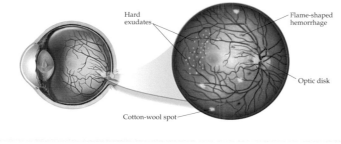

Hard exudates
Flame-shaped hemorrhage
Optic disk
Cotton-wool spot

Blood Vessel

Arteriosclerosis and Atherosclerosis

Sustained hypertension damages blood vessels. If blood vessels are subjected to high blood pressure for an extended period of time, they can thicken and harden, making them less flexible. This condition is called arteriosclerosis. Also, if excessive amounts of fat are found in the blood, the arteries can accumulate fatty deposits called plaques. This buildup, called atherosclerosis, causes the vessels to narrow or become obstructed.

Normal vessel   Arteriosclerosis   Atherosclerosis

Kidney

Nephrosclerosis

Nephrosclerosis is a kidney disorder in which the smallest arteries in the kidneys, called the arterioles, are damaged. Long-term hypertension causes the walls of the small blood vessels in the kidney to harden (arteriosclerosis). Over time, this causes a decrease in the blood flow to the kidneys and eventually causes the kidneys to scar and fail. This may lead to a need for kidney dialysis, in which a machine filters waste products from the blood for the kidneys, or a kidney transplant.

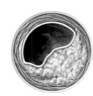

Glomerulus
Arteriosclerosis

Heart

Aortic Aneurysm

The aorta is the largest blood vessel in the body. It comes out of the top of the heart and brings blood to the rest of the body. Long-term high blood pressure can cause the wall of the aorta to weaken and balloon out (aneurysm). The aorta is then at risk of sudden rupture or tear, often leading to death.

Myocardial Infarction (Heart attack)

Myocardial infarction, or heart attack, results from narrowing or blockage (atherosclerosis) of one or more of the coronary arteries. This deprives the heart of oxygen, resulting in myocardial ischemia (disruption of the blood supply), infarction (tissue damage), and injury.

Left Ventricular Hypertrophy (LVH)

The muscle of the heart's left ventricle may become thickened and enlarged (LVH) due to long-term hypertension. The heart then becomes less efficient at circulating blood throughout the body. The resulting condition is called congestive heart failure. This may cause the lungs to fill up with fluid, resulting in difficulty breathing, fluid retention and swollen legs, and decreased blood flow to various parts of the body.

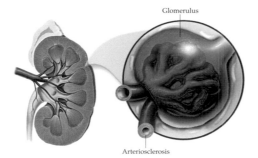
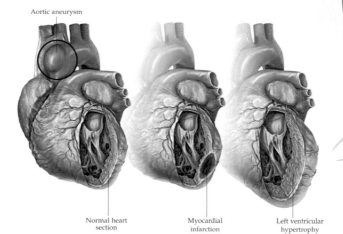

Aortic aneurysm
Normal heart section   Myocardial infarction   Left ventricular hypertrophy

Brain
Blood vessel
Lung
Heart
Lung
Liver
Spleen
Kidney
Kidney

49

Understanding Influenza

What Is Influenza?

Influenza, also known as the flu, is caused by the influenza virus. It is a contagious infection of the nose, throat, and lungs.

Influenza virus spreads in the little drops that spray out of an infected person's mouth and nose when he sneezes, coughs, laughs, or even talks.

When someone else breathes in these drops or gets them on his hands and then touches his own mouth or nose, the virus can enter his body .

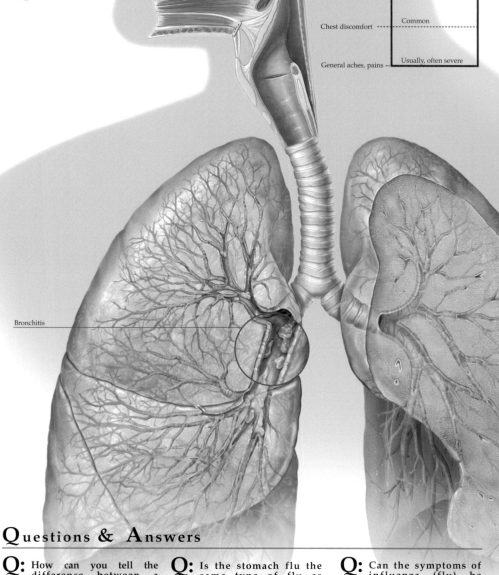

Flu Symptoms

Headache	Almost always
Fever	Usually high 102-104 F or 38.9-40 C
Fatigue, weakness	Can last up to two to three weeks
Runny or stuffy nose	Sometimes
Sneezing	Sometimes
Sore throat	Sometimes
Cough	Can become severe
Chest discomfort	Common
General aches, pains	Usually, often severe

Bronchitis

Prevention

Ways to Help Prevent Influenza

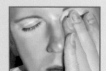

Avoid touching your eyes, nose, and mouth.

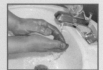

Wash your hands with soap and water frequently.

Get a vaccination (flu shot) every year before the start of the flu season. *Note: The vaccine does not cause the flu.*

Ways to Help Prevent the Spread of Influenza

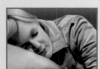

Stay home when you are sick.

Avoid close contact with others.

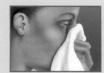

Cover your mouth and nose with a tissue when coughing or sneezing.

Special Risk Factors

Certain people have an increased risk of serious complications from influenza:
• People age 65 years and older
• People of any age with chronic medical conditions
• Pregnant women
• Children between 6 months and 23 months of age

Flu Vaccination (Flu Shot)

Because the influenza virus is different every year, you should protect yourself by getting a flu shot every year. If you are at high risk for major complications from the flu, it is especially important to get the shot before the flu season. The influenza vaccine may also lessen the severity of symptoms related to other forms of influenza that the vaccine is unable to prevent. The flu shot will not protect you from the common cold.

Complications

The complications caused by influenza include:
• Bacterial pneumonia
• Dehydration
• Worsening of chronic medical conditions, such as congestive heart failure, asthma, or diabetes
• Children may develop sinus problems or ear infections

Most people who get influenza recover in one to two weeks, but some people develop life-threatening complications (such as pneumonia) as a result of the flu. If your flu symptoms are unusually severe , you should seek medical help immediately.

Bronchitis, or inflammation of the bronchi, is another complication of influenza. In most cases, it involves the large and medium-sized bronchi. In children, older people, and those with lung disease, the infection may spread and inflame the bronchioles or lung tissue.

What to Do If You Get Sick

If you develop an influenza infection, you should:
• Get plenty of rest
• Drink plenty of liquids
• Avoid using alcohol and tobacco

You can also take medications to relieve flu symptoms but never give aspirin to children or teenagers who have cold or flu symptoms without first speaking to your healthcare provider. Antiviral medications have been approved for treatment of influenza but must be prescribed by a doctor. There is no cure for the flu. The antiviral medications can help reduce the severity and the duration of the symptoms.

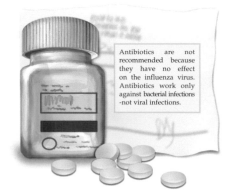

Antibiotics are not recommended because they have no effect on the influenza virus. Antibiotics work only against bacterial infections -not viral infections.

Questions & Answers

Q: How can you tell the difference between a common cold and influenza ?

A: Although flu and cold symptoms can be similar, the intensity and duration are different. The symptoms of a cold may come on gradually and are milder than the symptoms of the flu. Flu symptoms are more severe and tend to come on immediately and take longer to recover.

Q: Is the stomach flu the same type of flu as influenza (flu)?

A: No. Some people use the term "stomach flu" to describe certain common illnesses that can cause nausea, vomiting, or diarrhea. Although these symptoms can sometimes be related to the flu (more commonly in children), these problems are rarely symptoms of influenza.

Q: Can the symptoms of influenza (flu) be different in children?

A: Yes. Although flu symptoms for children and adults might be similar, children might have other symptoms such as nausea, vomiting and/or diarrhea. Children are at a higher risk of complications from the flu. If a child's symptoms worsen, call your doctor.

©2008 Wolters Kluwer Health | Lippincott Williams & Wilkins I Published by Anatomical Chart Company, Skokie, IL

50

Understanding Lung Cancer

Lung cancer is the rapid growth of abnormal (malignant) cells in one or both of the lungs. It can invade nearby tissues and may spread (metastasize) to other areas of the body.

Trachea

Lymph nodes

Metastasis to paratracheal lymph nodes

Bronchus

Tumor projecting into bronchi

Metastasis to carinal lymph nodes

LEFT UPPER LOBE

Tumor projecting into bronchi

LEFT LOWER LOBE

APPROXIMATELY 90% OF LUNG CANCER DEATHS ARE RELATED TO SMOKING

There are 2 Major Types of Lung Cancer: Non-Small Cell Lung Cancer and Small Cell Lung Cancer

Non-small cell lung cancer (NSCLC) is more common than small cell lung cancer, accounting for about 85% of all lung cancers; it generally grows and spreads more slowly. The three most common type of non-small cell lung cancer are:

1. **Adenocarcinoma** are the most common sub-type of NSCLC. It is usually found in the outer part of the lung.
2. **Squamous cell carcinoma** are tumors found near a bronchus.
3. **Large cell carcinoma** is a fast-growing form that can develop in any part of the lung.

NSCLC is staged according to the size of the tumor, the level of lymph node involvement, and the extent to which the cancer has spread. Stages include:

Stage 0	Cancer is limited to the lining of the air passages and has not yet invaded the lung tissue.
Stage I	Cancer has invaded the underlying lung tissue, but has not yet spread to the lymph nodes.
Stage II	Cancer has spread to the neighboring lymph nodes or have spread to the chest wall, or the diaphragm, or the pleura between the lungs, or membranes surrounding the heart.
Stage III	Cancer has spread from the lung to either the lymph nodes in the center of the chest or the collarbone area. The cancer may have spread locally to areas such as the heart, blood, vessels, trachea, and esophagus.
Stage IV	Cancer has spread to other parts of the body, such as the liver, bones, or brain.

Small cell lung cancer (SCLC), also known as oat cell cancer, is the less common form of lung cancer. It is a fast-growing cancer that forms in the tissues of the lungs and spreads to other parts of the body.

SCLC is staged differently from non-small cell types. Rather than using numbers, it is classified as either limited or extensive.

Limited	Cancer is confined to one lung and to its neighboring lymph nodes.
Extensive	Cancer has spread beyond one lung and nearby lymph nodes; it may have invaded both lungs, more remote lymph nodes, or other organs.

How is Lung Cancer Diagnosed?

The tests used to diagnose whether a patient has lung cancer varies depending on the patient's symptoms.

Chest X-Ray – Most patients under go this test to see if there are any abnormalities.

Chest CT Scan – If an abnormality is discovered in the chest x-ray, a computerized tomography (CT) scan is performed to provide a series of detailed pictures of parts inside the body, taken from different angles.

Biopsy – There are several different types of biopsy procedures. The choice of procedure, which may involve surgery, will depend on what is discovered via the chest x-ray and/or chest CT scan.

Sputum Cytology – A sample of phlegm is examined under a microscope.

CHEST X-RAY **CT SCAN** **PET SCAN** **MRI**

How is Lung Cancer Staged?

If cancer is diagnosed, more tests are done so the doctor can plan a treatment. These tests help discover the stage (extent) of the cancer. Common tests include:

Positron Emission Tomography (PET) scan – After a small amount of radioactive glucose (sugar) is injected into a vein of a patient, a special camera makes computerized pictures highlighting potential cancer cells.

PET/CT Scan – PET scan information is combined with the anatomical information from a CT scan to reliably determine whether an abnormal growth is cancerous or benign (non-cancerous).

Magnetic Resonance Imaging (MRI) of the Head – A powerful magnet linked to a computer produces detailed images of the areas inside the head.

Mediastinoscopy/Mediastinotomy – A lighted instrument (scope) is inserted into the body to examine the chest and nearby lymph nodes.

Risk Factors

- Smoking cigarettes, cigars, and pipes
- Exposure to:
  - Secondhand smoke
  - Radon – Radioactive gas that occurs naturally in soil and rocks. Mine workers may be exposed to radon. Radon may also be found in homes and buildings
  - Asbestos – Group of naturally-occurring fibrous minerals that are used in certain industries.
  - Pollution
- Having previous lung diseases, such at tuberculosis (TB) and emphysema
- Personal history – A person with a history of lung cancer is more likely to develop it again than someone who has never had the disease.
- Heredity – Genetics seem to play a role in who develops lung cancer

Signs and Symptoms

- Cough that does not go away
- Constant chest pain
- Coughing up blood
- Shortness of breath, wheezing, or hoarseness
- Problems with pneumonia or bronchitis
- Swelling of the neck and face
- Loss of appetite and/or weight
- Fatigue

If lung cancer has spread to other organs (metastasized), signs may include headaches, visual changes, stroke-like symptoms (if cancer has spread to the brain), and bone pain (if the cancer has spread to the bones).

Treatment Options

Treatment depends on a number of factors including the type of lung cancer, the size/location/stage of the tumor, and the general health and pulmonary function of the patient. Many different types of treatments or combination of treatments may be used, such as:

Surgical Resection – A portion of the lung containing the tumor is removed. Depending on the case, the surgeon may remove only a small portion, the entire lobe (lobectomy), or the entire lung (pneumonectomy). Lymph nodes are also sampled at the time of surgery. Lobectomy is the most widely used surgical procedure for lung cancer.

Chemotherapy – The use of anticancer drugs that kill cancer cells throughout the body.

Radiation therapy – The use of high-energy rays to kill cancer cells. This therapy is directed to a limited area and affects the cancer cells only in that area.

Endobronchial Therapy – A group of therapies used to treat lesions that are accessible in the lung airways. They are primarily used for palliative therapy (to relieve symptoms, not to cure the disease), but may also be used for early stages of the disease.

How can Lung Cancer be Prevented?

- **Don't smoke** – If you do smoke, quit. If you stop smoking, the risk of lung cancer decreases each year as normal cells replace abnormal cells. After 10 years, the risk drops to a level that is one-third to one-half of the risk of people who continue to smoke.
- **Avoid secondhand smoke**
- **Test your home for radon**
- **Avoid carcinogens** - People who are exposed to large amounts of asbestos should use protective equipment.

51

Understanding Menopause

What Is Perimenopause?

The time period during which certain events occur leading up to and following menopause is referred to as perimenopause. Perimenopause is the time in a woman's life from the first sign of menstrual irregularity to one year after the last menstrual period. The perimenopausal time is associated with many physical, emotional, and mental changes.

What Is Menopause?

The word *menopause* is derived from the Greek words *men*, which means "monthly," and *pauses*, which means "ending." Menopause is the date that marks a woman's last menstrual period. This end to the menstrual cycle means the end of ovulation, the end of menstrual periods, and the end of the possibility of pregnancy.

What Is Estrogen?

Estrogen is a hormone, a chemical substance secreted into body fluids that exerts an effect on specific cells of the body. The main source of estrogen during a woman's reproductive years is her ovaries.

Estrogen production goes down as the number of follicles decreases. When estrogen levels fall below a critical value, ovulation cannot occur consistently, and menstrual periods become irregular. Eventually, all follicles degenerate and reproductive cycles stop altogether.

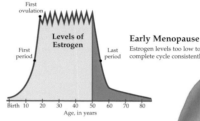

Early Menopause
Estrogen levels too low to complete cycle consistently.

What Are the Signs of Menopause?

While some menopausal women notice no changes other than the cessation of menstrual periods, others go through a variety of physical and/or emotional changes.

During menopause, estrogen production decreases; postmenopausal estrogen levels are about 75 percent lower than during the reproductive years. Changes experienced during perimenopause and menopause are the body's response to this decrease.

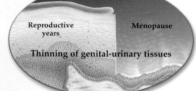

Hot Flashes, Night Sweats, and Insomnia

Hot flashes are characterized by redness and/or sweating in the face, neck, and chest. Hot flash symptoms may happen throughout the day and night (night sweats), causing discomfort and interfering with restful sleep.

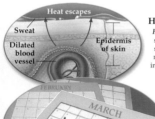

Irregular Menstruation

Irregular periods (perimenopause) or *no periods* (menopause). Irregularity of menstrual periods is the earliest, most common symptom of menopause. Once you experience a six-month lapse in menstrual periods, there is a 90 percent chance that menstruation will not resume.

Painful Intercourse

Thinning of genital-urinary tissues may lead to painful intercourse.

Reproductive years — **Menopause**
Thinning of genital-urinary tissues

Emotional/Mental Signs
- Fatigue caused by sleep deprivation.
- Mood disturbances.
- Forgetfulness.
- Decreased sex drive.
- Depression.
- Nervousness.

Other Signs
- Muscle and joint pain.
- Backaches.
- Headaches.
- Dizziness.
- Urinary incontinence.
- Prickling or itching sensations of the skin.
- Palpitations (periods of rapid heartbeat).

No Signs
Some women experience no symptoms other than cessation of menstrual periods.

Although all of these occurrences are normal, it is important to see your doctor regularly to discuss your symptoms.

What Changes Might I Expect?

Hair Growth
- Thinning of scalp hair.
- Darkening or thickening of other body hair, such as facial hair.

Skin
- Loss of firmness, tension, and fluid.
- Decrease in melanocytes, which give skin pigment.
- Increased sensitivity to sun exposure.

Bone
- Becomes progressively more porous and brittle.
- Increased risk of osteoporosis.
- More subject to fractures.

Circulatory System
- Increased heart disease risk.
- Increased high blood pressure risk.
- Increased high cholesterol risk.

Breasts
- Less firm breasts. Glandular tissue is replaced with fat.

Reproductive System
- Few remaining follicles (egg cells) in ovaries.
- Reproductive organs decrease in size.
- Vaginal mucosa become thinner, less lubricated.
- Vaginal pH changes, increasing susceptibility to infection.
- Endometriosis disappears.

Urinary System
- Thinning of tissues in bladder and urethra.
- Increased risk of urinary tract infections.

Another health concern associated with menopause is weight gain.

The Ovary and Its Role in Reproduction and Menopause

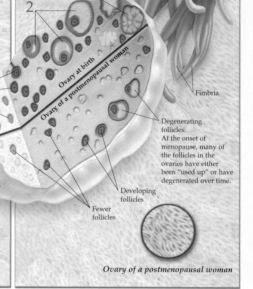

Egg Development During Reproductive Years

1. After the onset of puberty, about 20 *follicles* (egg cells) begin to develop each month and secrete estrogen.

2. Estrogen stimulates further *enlargement of the follicles* until one outgrows the other and releases an egg into the fallopian tube. This is called ovulation.

3. The empty follicle is called the *corpus luteum*, which mainly secretes progesterone, that stabilizes the endometrial lining. If pregnancy does not occur, the corpus luteum starts to degenerate, the lining is "less stable" and a period occurs. Estrogen is secreted from the follicle prior to ovulation. After ovulation, progesterone is its main hormone, but smaller amounts of estrogen are also secreted.

Degenerating follicles: At the onset of menopause, many of the follicles in the ovaries have either been "used up" or have degenerated over time.

Ovary: The two ovaries contain 700,000 follicles, or egg cells, at birth.

Ovary at birth

Ovary of a postmenopausal woman

Is Hormone Replacement Therapy (HRT) Right for Me?

Menopause is a natural part of a woman's life cycle. However, it is a time when a woman can make several health-related decisions. Hormone replacement therapy (HRT) has been shown to reduce the risk of osteoporosis and colon cancer, but may increase the risk of breast cancer, heart disease, stroke, and blood clots. Deciding whether to take postmenopausal hormone replacement is complicated for many women. The benefits of hormone replacement therapy are significant, but they must be weighed against the potential risks. Women should consult with their physician about HRT to determine if it is appropriate for them.

Some of the factors associated with HRT:

Benefits	Risks
• Reduced osteoporosis risk. • Reduced incontinence risk. • Decreased vaginal dryness and irritation. • Decreased hot flashes. • Increased energy. • Decreased risk of colon cancer. • Improved memory.	• Increased risk of endometrial cancer (if using unopposed Estrogen). • Increased risk of stroke. • Increased risk of blood clots. • Possible increased risk of gallbladder disease. • Possible increased risk of heart disease. • Possible increased risk of breast cancer. • Other potential side effects: Bloating, fluid retention, breast tenderness, headaches, mood changes, and nausea.

regular doctor visits

HRT medications

How Can I Take Charge of My Health?

Whether you choose to take *HRT* or not, consider other options. This is a great time to *re-establish a relationship with a health care provider*. Women should take advantage of preventive options such as:

- *regular breast exams*
- *mammograms*
- *colonoscopies*
- *bloodwork to check thyroid function and lipid profile*
- *regular exercise**
- *eat a healthy diet that is high in fiber and calcium and low in fat*

**Be sure to engage in weight-bearing exercise, such as walking or jogging, several times a week to slow the loss of bone mass.*

breast self exams

mammograms

thyroid and cholesterol checks

healthy diet

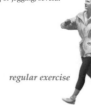

regular exercise

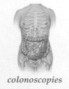

colonoscopies

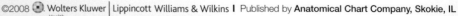

How Pain Works

3 Brain processes the message and alerts the body of pain.

Brain

Spinal cord

Nerves

2 Nerves pick up the injury and send the message to the brain.

- *Red dashed line show message flow from pain site to brain.*
- *Blue dotted line show message going from brain to pain site.*

1 Injury occurs in the body.

What Is Pain?

It is an unpleasant sensation occurring in varying degrees of severity associated with injury, disease, or emotional disorder.

2 Types of Pain

1. ACUTE PAIN

occurs as a result of injury to the body and generally disappears when the physical injury heals. Acute pain is linked to tissue injury. Anxiety is common with acute pain.

Examples include:
- Surgical pain
- Muscle strains
- Orthopedic-type injuries
- Labor and delivery

Symptoms: Patient is able to point to site of pain.
- Sharp
- Burning
- Cramping
- Aching
- Pressured

2. CHRONIC (PERSISTENT) PAIN

lasts beyond the normal healing period – usually at least 3 months. The pain may be multifocal and vague. There may be no signs on x-rays or scans to indicate the source of the pain since some pain may be generated by tissue injury. Depression is common with chronic pain.

Neuropathic chronic pain is a type of pain that is caused by injury to a nerve. Patients describe the pain as having tingling, numbness, or burning sensation. Neuropathic pain is difficult to treat.

Common types of neuropathic chronic pain include:
- Diabetic neuropathy – nerve damage as a result of high blood sugar.
- Post-herpetic neuralgia – pain from shingles after the blisters have healed.
- HIV/AIDS – pain from the viral illness or the drugs used to treat the disease.
- Peripheral vascular disease – pain in legs, usually during activity, from lack of blood supply to the extremities. The legs may be discolored, cold, and the skin may be shiny.

Symptoms:
- Painful itching
- Strange sensations
- Extreme sensitivity to normal touch and temperature
- Burning
- Electric-like sensation
- Painful numbness
- Pins and needles

Non-neuropathic chronic pain is pain that is not caused by injury to a nerve.

The most common types include:
- Low back pain – pain in the lower back from muscles, ligaments, tendons, arthritis, or damaged discs.
- Osteoarthritis – arthritis resulting from wear and tear of the joints and with normal aging.
- Rheumatoid arthritis – an autoimmune disorder resulting in pain, stiffness, and inflammation of the joints.

Symptoms: Poorly localized pain (patient may not be able to point to site of pain).
- Gnawing
- Pounding
- Deep aching

Unknown: There are many common chronic pain syndromes that are neither known to be chronic non-neuropathic nor neuropathic.

These include:
- Fibromyalgia syndrome – diffuse body pain with tenderness in the muscles.
- Tension headache – pressure-type headache lasting days to weeks and often not severe.
- Migraine headache – episodic headache that persists for hours to days with nausea and is often severe.
- Irritable bowel syndrome (IBS) – abdominal pain with cramping, bloating, and constipation often alternating with diarrhea.
- Some low back pain – back pain that is not muscular, not related to disc injury, and without a known cause.

Symptoms: May be a combination of chronic non-neuropathic and neuropathic symptoms.

Treatment

Specific treatment options need to be tailored to the individual patient. Be sure to consult with your healthcare professional to determine the right treatment for you.

Prevention techniques:
- Regular exercise • Maintain a healthy body weight • Use safe techniques when lifting heavy objects

Where do you Feel Pain?

Right   Left

Left   Right

Pain Scale

0 1 2 3 4 5 6 7 8 9 10

No pain   *Rate your pain by choosing the number that best describes it.*   *Extreme pain*

53

Sexually Transmitted Infections

What Are Sexually Transmitted Infections?

Sexually transmitted infections (STIs) are diseases you can get by having sex with someone who has an infection. There are more than 20 types of STIs, which can be spread during vaginal, oral, and anal sexual contact. STIs can be painful, and may have serious consequences (including death) if not treated. **Bacterial** STIs like gonorrhea and chlamydia are relatively easy to cure if treated early, but **viral** STIs, like genital herpes and the human immunodeficiency virus (HIV) cannot be cured. Other STIs such as trichomoniasis are caused by **protozoa** (single-celled organisms), and **parasites** are responsible for pubic lice and scabies.

Complications

Without treatment, sexually transmitted infections can lead to serious health problems— especially in women. In addition, STIs increase the risk of acquiring and transmitting HIV, the virus that causes AIDS. Some complications of STIs and the organs affected are listed below:

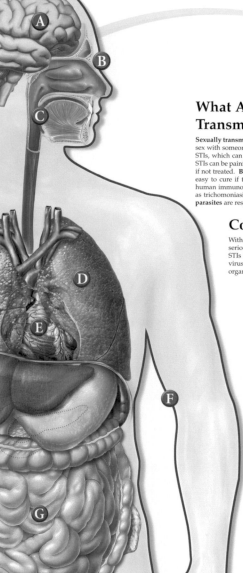

(A) Brain and Nervous System - Headaches, brain damage, meningitis (inflamed lining of the brain), stroke, neurological disorders (nervous system problems), psychiatric illness, spinal damage

(B) Eyes - Conjunctivitis, blindness

(C) Mouth and Throat - Thrush (infection of the oral tissues), pharyngitis (inflamed throat)

(D) Lungs - Peumocystis carinii (form of pneumonia common in people with reduced immunity)

(E) Heart and Blood Vessels - Aortic stenosis (narrowing of artery and/or valve of the heart), inflammation of the aorta, aneurysm (bulging) of the aorta, Kaposi's sarcoma (AIDS-related cancer affecting walls of certain lymphatic vessels)

(F) Skin - Rashes, itching, blisters, ulcers

(G) Intestines - Dysentery (inflammation of the intestine, with abdominal pain and frequent, watery stools)

(H) Urinary System - Cystitis (inflammation of the bladder), urinary tract infections, urethritis (inflammation of urethra)

(I) Bones and Joints - Arthritis, bone aches

Reproductive system complications include:

Male– Prostatitis (inflammation of the prostate gland), sterility, impotence, epididymitis (inflammation of the epididymis), urethral stricture

Female– Pelvic scarring, genital damage, cervical cancer, infertility, vulvovaginitis (inflammation of vulva and vagina), ectopic (tubal) pregnancy

Signs and Symptoms

The table below lists some of the most common symptoms of STIs. It is important to remember that many women and men who have an STI often do not experience any symptoms at all. If you are experiencing any of the symptoms listed below or if you believe you have an STI, talk to your health care provider as soon as possible.

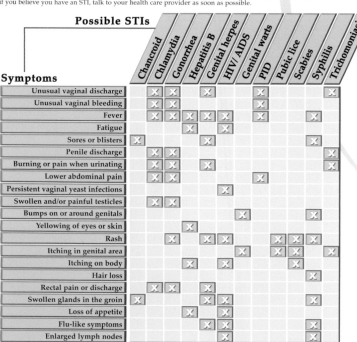

Possible STIs

Symptoms	Chancroid	Chlamydia	Gonorrhea	Hepatitis B	Genital herpes	HIV/AIDS	Genital warts	PID	Pubic lice	Scabies	Syphilis	Trichomoniasis
Unusual vaginal discharge		X	X		X		X					X
Unusual vaginal bleeding		X	X				X					
Fever	X	X	X	X	X	X					X	
Fatigue				X		X						
Sores or blisters	X				X						X	
Penile discharge		X	X									X
Burning or pain when urinating		X	X		X							X
Lower abdominal pain	X	X	X					X				
Persistent vaginal yeast infections						X						
Swollen and/or painful testicles		X	X									
Bumps on or around genitals							X				X	
Yellowing of eyes or skin				X								
Rash		X		X	X	X			X	X	X	
Itching in genital area					X		X		X	X		X
Itching on body				X		X				X		
Hair loss											X	
Rectal pain or discharge		X	X		X							
Swollen glands in the groin	X										X	
Loss of appetite			X	X								
Flu-like symptoms				X	X							X
Enlarged lymph nodes				X								X

Genital Warts

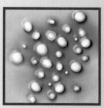

Genital warts are painless growths found on or around the genital and anal areas. They are caused by the human papillomavirus (HPV). Despite treatment, genital warts cannot be cured and often recur. In women, infection with certain strains of HPV can increase the risk of developing cervical cancer.

Genital Herpes

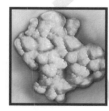

Genital herpes is a viral infection that causes painful sores on and around the genitals or anal area. It is easily spread and the disease tends to recur, especially in the first few years after initial infection. There is no cure, but there are medications that can help relieve symptoms.

Chancroid

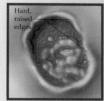

Soft, ragged edges
Pus

Chancroid (shan-kroid) is a bacterial infection that causes painful ulcers on the genitals. The chancroid ulcer can be difficult to distinguish from ulcers that are caused by genital herpes and syphilis. Symptoms usually appear within a week of exposure.

Syphilis

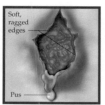

Hard, raised edges

Syphilis is a bacterial infection, that can damage organs over time if untreated. The first symptom of syphilis is an ulcer called a **chancre** (shan-ker). Left untreated, about one-third of cases will go onto the later, more damaging, stages.

Trichomoniasis

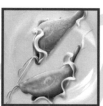

One of the most common STIs, trichomoniasis (trick-oh-moh-nye-uh-sis) is a genital-tract infection caused by a protozoan (single-celled organism). This STI is usually transmitted through sexual intercourse, but a woman can also transmit the infection to her baby during childbirth.

HIV/AIDS

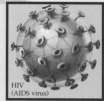

HIV (AIDS virus)

HIV (human immuno-deficiency virus) infects and gradually destroys cells in the immune system. HIV severely weakens the body's response to infections and cancers. Eventually, AIDS (acquired immunodeficiency syndrome) is diagnosed. With AIDS, a variety of infections can overtake the body and eventually cause death.

Pelvic Inflammatory Disease (PID)

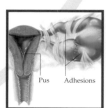

Pus   Adhesions

PID is a term used to describe an infection of the uterus, fallopian tubes or ovaries. It is the most common, serious infection among young women. PID infection can cause scarring of the tissue inside the fallopian tubes, which can damage the tubes or block them completely. If untreated, PID can result in infertility, ectopic pregnancy, miscarriage, or chronic pain.

Hepatitis B

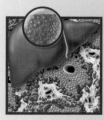

The liver disease Hepatitis B is caused by a virus carried in the blood, saliva, semen, and other body fluids of an infected person. It is spread through sexual contact and can be spread from a mother to her baby during childbirth or during breastfeeding. Recovery usually happens within six months, but in rare cases hepatitis B can lead to liver damage and an increased risk of liver cancer.

Pubic Lice

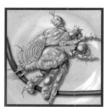

Pubic lice are tiny parasites that live in pubic hair and survive by feeding on human blood. They are most often spread by sexual activity, but in rare cases they can be spread through contact with infested clothing or bedding. It is unusual for pubic lice to cause any serious health problems, but the itching they cause can be very uncomfortable.

Scabies

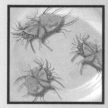

Scabies is a parasitic skin infection caused by a tiny mite. Highly contagious, it is spread primarily through sexual contact, though it also can be spread through contact with skin, infested clothing, or bedding. Scabies causes intense itching, which often is worse at night.

Chlamydia

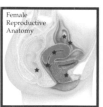

Female Reproductive Anatomy

Chlamydia is a bacterial infection very similar to gonorrhea. Up to 50 percent of men, and 75 percent of women don't experience any symptoms. Complications for women are more serious than for men. In women chlamydia can cause irreversible damage, such as pelvic inflammatory disease and infertility.

★ = sites of chlamydia and gonorrhea infection

Gonorrhea

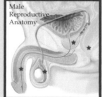

Male Reproductive Anatomy

Gonorrhea, is a curable STI which can infect the genital tract, the mouth, and the rectum. It is usually spread through sexual contact, but an infected woman can pass the disease to her baby during delivery. Often there are no symptoms. Untreated it can cause sterility in both sexes.

★ = sites of chlamydia and gonorrhea infection

Prevention and Treatment

The only way to eliminate the risk of acquiring an STI is to avoid sex *completely*. But there are several measures you can take to *reduce* your risk and to avoid transmitting STIs:

- Avoid sex with multiple partners.
- Use a condom.
- Get a Hepatitis B immunization (shot).
- Become familiar with the symptoms of STIs.
- Know your sexual partner's sexual history.

- Have regular checkups for STIs, even if you have no symptoms.
- Seek medical help immediately if any suspicious symptoms develop.

- If infected, tell any past or present partner(s) so that they may get treated.
- Avoid all sexual activity while being treated for an STI.

Most STIs are easily treated. The earlier a person seeks treatment, the less likely the disease will cause permanent physical damage, be spread to others, or be passed on from a mother to her newborn baby.

54

Understanding Sleep Disorders

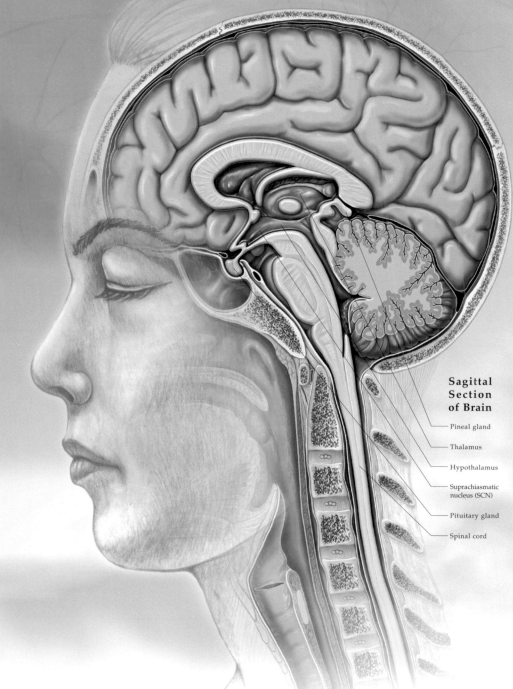

Sagittal Section of Brain

- Pineal gland
- Thalamus
- Hypothalamus
- Suprachiasmatic nucleus (SCN)
- Pituitary gland
- Spinal cord

What Is Sleep?

Sleep is a natural, reversible state of decreased responsiveness to the environment. During sleep, usually the eyes are closed and the body is relaxed and almost motionless. We think of sleep in contrast to wakefulness, when the body and mind are active. Although sleep provides important rest and restoration for the brain and body, the brain is very active during the portions of sleep when we are dreaming.

Why Does the Body Need Sleep?

Sleep is important for survival and appears to have specific functions for the endocrine, immune, cardiovascular, and nervous systems. It also has been suggested that sleep is important for bodily restoration, energy conservation, and memory consolidation. Not having an appropriate amount of normal, restful sleep may seriously affect daily functioning.

What Does the Suprachiasmatic Nucleus (SCN) Do?

The suprachiasmatic nucleus (SCN) is an area of the hypothalamus that initiates signals to other parts of the brain that control hormones, body temperature, and other functions that play a role in making you feel sleepy or wide awake. The SCN works like a biological clock that sets off a regulated pattern of activities that affect the whole body. The SCN controls the production of melatonin in the pineal gland. During the day the melatonin level is very low, but it increases in the evening and is elevated throughout the night, when you normally sleep. The functioning of the SCN normally helps you sleep for about 8 hours at night and remain awake for about 16 hours in the daytime and evening.

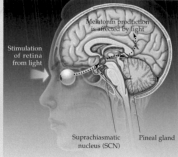

Melatonin production is affected by light

Stimulation of retina from light

Suprachiasmatic nucleus (SCN)

Pineal gland

Stages of Sleep

People usually cycle through different stages of sleep. Time spent in these stages may vary with age.

Non-REM *75–80% of sleep*	As you fall asleep, you enter non-REM sleep, which comprises of *Stages 1 – 4* *
*Stage 1 ***	Drowsiness and light sleep.
*Stage 2 ***	This stage takes up a majority of a night's total sleep. It is defined by unique EEG characteristics.
*Stages 3 & 4 ***	Deepest and most restorative sleep: Blood pressure drops, breathing slows down, and hormones are released for growth and development in youths.
REM *(Rapid Eye Movement)* *20–25% of sleep*	Occurs in episodes beginning about 90 minutes after onset of sleep and recurring with lengthening episodes about every 90 minutes. Most REM sleep is during the latter half of the night. The brain is active and dreams occur as the eyes dart back and forth. The body becomes relaxed and immobile. Breathing and heart rate may become irregular.

Normal Sleep Pattern

Awake / REM / Stage 1 / 2 / 3 / 4

Hours 1 2 3 4 5 6 7 8

Tips for a Good Night's Sleep

- Try to keep a regular bedtime and wakeup time.
- Avoid napping if you can't sleep well at night.
- Don't lie in bed awake if you can't sleep.
- Try to relax before going to bed.
- Exercise regularly, but not close to bedtime.
- Avoid caffeine, nicotine, and alcohol before bed.
- Maintain a comfortable room temperature.
- See a doctor if sleep problems continue.

Common Sleep Disorders

Sleep disorders can interfere with the ability to sleep or remain awake at the appropriate times. Some sleep disorders involve behaviors or experiences that occur in association with sleep. Some of the most common sleep disorders are shown below.

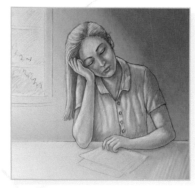

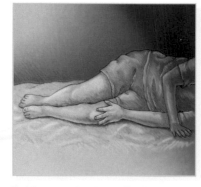

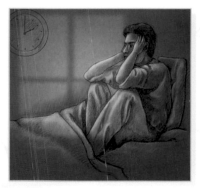

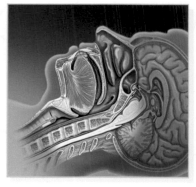

Narcolepsy

People with narcolepsy feel sleepy throughout their waking time, in spite of having sufficient opportunity for sleep at nighttime. They may nap several times a day but feel refreshed only for short periods. At times, sleep seems irresistible. They often have problems concentrating. Inattention and sleepiness can interfere with normal daily functioning. People with narcolepsy may experience cataplexy (*sudden muscle weakness during emotional situations*) and, when falling asleep, a brief sense of muscle paralysis or dreamlike hallucinations.

Restless Legs Syndrome (RLS)

Restless legs syndrome (RLS) is a disorder that causes a very unpleasant crawling sensation, mostly in the legs. The natural response is an urge to move them for relief. It usually is worst in the evening and when someone is at rest. It often interferes with the ability to sleep and may cause involuntary kicking during sleep. Someone with severe RLS may feel very uncomfortable sitting for a prolonged period of time in a theater or riding long distances in a car. Restless legs syndrome symptoms can begin at any age.

Insomnia

Insomnia is the most common sleep problem. It may include difficulty falling asleep and staying asleep, as well as a sense of light or unrefreshing sleep. Most commonly it is due to stress, but it also may result from psychiatric (*mental*), medical, and other sleep disorders. Poor sleep habits can contribute to insomnia. For most people, insomnia lasts just a few days or weeks, but for others it may be a chronic condition lasting years. The daytime consequences are fatigue, lack of energy, difficulty concentrating, and irritability.

Obstructive Sleep Apnea

Obstructive sleep apnea is a recurrent interruption in breathing during sleep. It results from sleep-related muscle relaxation in the upper airway, which leads to a decrease or complete blockage of airflow for brief periods. The blood oxygen level may fall, causing arousals or awakenings that can disturb sleep. People with severe sleep apnea may be dangerously sleepy during the daytime. Those who are obese or snore loudly are at the greatest risk for sleep apnea, but others may have sleep apnea due to large tonsils or other features of their airway anatomy.

55

Understanding Stroke

What Is Stroke?

Stroke refers to the sudden death of brain tissue caused by a lack of oxygen resulting from an interrupted blood supply. An **infarct** is the area of the brain that has "died" because of this lack of oxygen. There are two ways that brain tissue death can occur. **Ischemic stroke** is a blockage or reduction of blood flow in an artery that feeds that area of the brain. It is the most common cause of an infarct. **Hemorrhagic stroke** results from bleeding within and around the brain causing compression and tissue injury.

Ischemic Stroke

This type of stroke results from a blockage or reduction of blood flow to an area of the brain. This blockage may result from atherosclerosis and blood clot formation.

Atherosclerosis is the deposit of cholesterol and plaque within the walls of arteries. These deposits may become large enough to narrow the lumen and reduce the flow of blood while also causing the artery to lose its ability to stretch.

A **thrombus**, or blood clot, forms on the roughened surface of atherosclerotic plaques that develop in the wall of the artery. The thrombus can enlarge and eventually block the lumen of the artery.

- Lumen
- Plaque
- Thrombus

Common Sites of Plaque Formation

(Indicated by yellow circles)

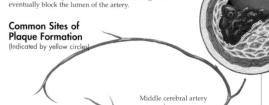

- Middle cerebral artery
- Posterior cerebral artery
- Anterior cerebral artery
- Anterior inferior cerebellar artery
- Posterior inferior cerebellar artery
- Embolus
- Internal carotid artery
- Embolus
- Vertebral artery
- Common carotid artery

Part of a thrombus may break off and become an **embolus**. An embolus travels through the blood stream until it reaches a vessel too small for it to pass through, thus blocking it.

Emboli commonly come from the heart, where different diseases can cause thrombus formation.

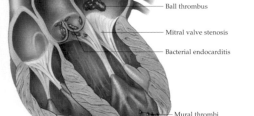

- Atrial fibrillation
- Ball thrombus
- Mitral valve stenosis
- Bacterial endocarditis
- Mural thrombi
- Myocardial infarction

Hemorrhagic Stroke

This type of stroke is caused by bleeding within and around the brain. Bleeding that fills the spaces between the brain and the skull is called a **subarachnoid hemorrhage**. It is caused by ruptured aneurysms, arteriovenous malformations, and head trauma. Bleeding within the brain tissue itself is known as **intracerebral hemorrhage** and is primarily caused by hypertension.

An **aneurysm** is a weakening of the arterial wall that causes it to stretch and balloon. It usually occurs where the artery branches.

Hypertension is an elevation of blood pressure that may cause tiny arterioles to burst causing the tissue beyond the rupture to die. Blood vessels in the dead tissue then leak causing more bleeding.

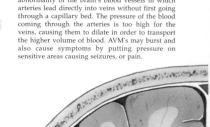

- Circle of Willis
- Aneurysm

An **arteriovenous malformation** (AVM) is an abnormality of the brain's blood vessels in which arteries lead directly into veins without first going through a capillary bed. The pressure of the blood coming through the arteries is too high for the veins, causing them to dilate in order to transport the higher volume of blood. AVM's may burst and also cause symptoms by putting pressure on sensitive areas causing seizures, or pain.

- Intracerebral hemorrhage
- Arteriovenous malformation (AVM)

- Subarachnoid hemorrhage
- Arterioles
- Microaneurysm

Normal Functional Areas of Brain

The brain has two sides: a right hemisphere that controls the left side of the body and a left hemisphere that controls the right side of the body. Each hemisphere has four lobes and a cerebellum that control our daily functions. Depending on what part of the brain has been affected, stroke victims experience a variety of neurological deficits. Rehabilitation is crucial to the stroke patient's recovery. Physical therapists and speech therapists help patients "relearn" their lost functions and devise ways to cope with the loss of those they cannot regain.

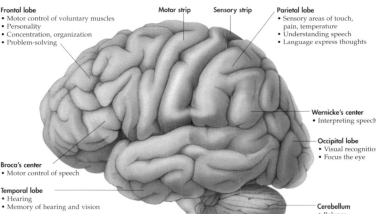

Frontal lobe
- Motor control of voluntary muscles
- Personality
- Concentration, organization
- Problem-solving

Motor strip **Sensory strip**

Parietal lobe
- Sensory areas of touch, pain, temperature
- Understanding speech
- Language express thoughts

Wernicke's center
- Interpreting speech

Occipital lobe
- Visual recognition
- Focus the eye

Broca's center
- Motor control of speech

Temporal lobe
- Hearing
- Memory of hearing and vision

Cerebellum
- Balance
- Coordinating muscle movement

Brain stem
- Controls heart rate and rate of breathing

Events Leading to Stroke

Stroke victims often have small strokes or "warning signs," before a large permanent attack.

Transient Ischemic Attacks (TIAs) are brief attacks that last anywhere from a few minutes to 24 hours. The symptoms resolve completely and the person returns to normal. It is possible to have several TIAs before a large attack.

Complete Infarction (CI) is an attack that leaves permanent tissue death and results in serious neurological deficits. Recovery is usually not total and takes longer than three weeks.

Common Neurological Deficits After Stroke

Left-sided stroke
- Right-sided paralysis
- Speech/language deficits
- Slow, cautious behavior
- Hemianopsia of right visual field
- Memory loss in language
- Right-sided dysarthria
- Aphasia
- Apraxia

Right-sided stroke
- Left-sided paralysis
- Spatial/perceptual deficits
- Quick, impulsive behavior
- Hemianopsia of left visual field
- Memory loss in performance
- Left-sided dysarthria

Related Terms

Paralysis - Loss of muscle function and sensation

Hemiparesis - Weakness of muscles on one side of body

Hemianopsia - Loss of sight in half of visual field

Aphasia - Difficulty with oral communication, reduced ability to read or write

Apraxia - Inability to control muscles; movement is uncoordinated and jerky

Dysarthria - Slurring of speech and "mouth droop" on one side of face due to muscle weakness

Risks for Stroke

- Hypertension
- Heart disease
- Atherosclerosis
- Previous TIAs
- High cholesterol
- High alcohol consumption
- Obesity
- Diabetes
- Bruit noise in carotid artery
- Cigarette smoking
- Oral contraceptive use
- Family history of stroke

Thyroid Disorders

56

What Is the Thyroid?

The thyroid is a small gland that is wrapped around the windpipe (trachea), just below the thyroid cartilage. The thyroid plays an important role in health and affects every organ, tissue, and cell in the body. It makes hormones that maintain the normal function of many organ systems and regulate metabolism (how the body uses and stores energy from foods eaten).

When the thyroid is not working properly (called thyroid disorder), it can affect:

- Body weight
- Energy level
- Sleeping patterns
- Skin & hair
- Fertility & menstruation
- Memory & concentration
- Bone strength
- Cholesterol level

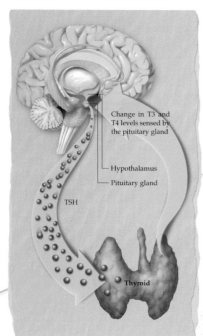

Normal Hormone Production

The thyroid gland is controlled by the pituitary gland. When the level of thyroid hormones (T3 & T4) drops too low, the pituitary gland responds by producing thyroid-stimulating hormone (TSH). TSH is a good marker of thyroid hormone balance: when the thyroid gland is underactive, TSH is high; when overactive, TSH is low.

Change in T3 and T4 levels sensed by the pituitary gland
Hypothalamus
Pituitary gland
TSH
Thyroid

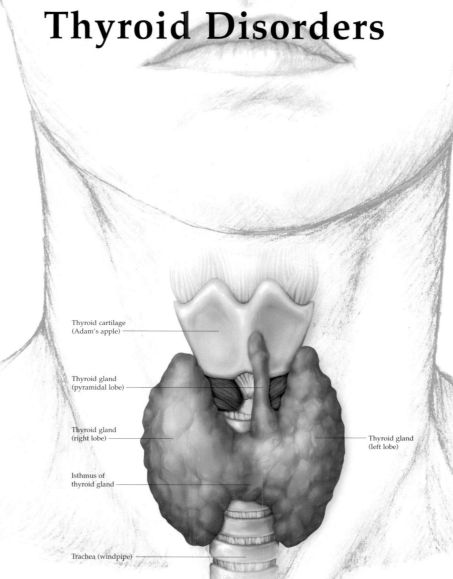

Thyroid cartilage (Adam's apple)
Thyroid gland (pyramidal lobe)
Thyroid gland (right lobe)
Thyroid gland (left lobe)
Isthmus of thyroid gland
Trachea (windpipe)

How to Check Your Thyroid

As a first step in identifying an underlying thyroid problem, you should do a simple thyroid self-exam.

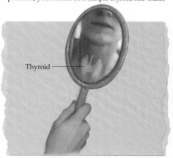

Thyroid

1. While holding a mirror, look at the area of your neck just below the Adam's apple. This is where you will find your thyroid.

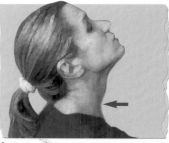

2. Tip your head back, while focusing on the thyroid area in the mirror.

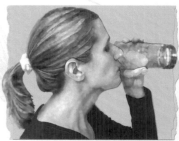

3. Take a drink of water. Look at your neck and check for any lumps in this area while you swallow.

Overactive Thyroid

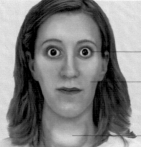

Broken lines indicate normal size of thyroid.

Bulging eyes
Face is thin from weight loss
Swelling of neck (goiter)

Common Thyroid Disorders

Overactive thyroid (hyperthyroidism):
When the thyroid gland is overactive, it makes too much of the thyroid hormone. This condition affects women more than men.

Graves' disease:
One of the most common causes of overactive thyroid, especially among women. It occurs when the immune system, which normally protects the body from bacteria and viruses, mistakenly attacks the thyroid gland and causes it to overproduce the thyroid hormone thyroxine. This autoimmune response can also affect the tissue behind the eyes (Graves' ophthalmopathy) and the skin on the shins (Graves' dermopathy).

Postpartum thyroiditis:
After childbirth, a woman's thyroid can become larger or inflamed. This condition usually goes away within six months, with no permanent damage to the thyroid.

Symptoms

- Sudden weight loss, even when appetite and food intake remain normal or increase.
- Rapid or irregular heartbeat or pounding of the heart.
- Nervousness, irritability, tremor.
- Sweating.
- Changes in menstrual patterns.
- Increased sensitivity to heat.
- Changes in bowel patterns, especially more frequent bowel movements.
- Enlarged thyroid (goiter), which may appear as a swelling at the base of the neck.
- Fatigue, muscle weakness.
- Difficulty sleeping.
- Pain or discomfort in the neck.

Underactive Thyroid

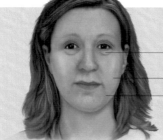

Broken lines indicate normal size of thyroid.

Puffiness under eyes
Puffy face
Dry skin

Underactive thyroid (hypothyroidism):
The most common type of thyroid disorder, where the thyroid makes too little of the thyroid hormone.

Hashimoto's disease:
The most often cause of underactive thyroid which can occur at any age but is most common in middle-aged and older women and in those who have a family history of this problem. It occurs when the immune system reacts against the thyroid gland, causing it to become inflamed (chronic thyroiditis).

Underactive thyroid and pregnancy:
A fetus depends on their mother's thyroid hormone for normal development. During pregnancy, women need more thyroid hormone, so thyroid testing is recommended every few weeks to ensure that the levels remain in balance.

- Increased sensitivity to cold.
- Constipation.
- Rough, cold, and dry skin.
- Puffy face.
- Hoarse voice.
- Poor concentration.
- Heavier-than-normal menstrual periods.
- Depression.
- Tingling sensations in legs and arms.
- Sleepiness.
- Unexplained weight gain.
Note: There may be no symptoms.

Thyroid Nodules and Cancer

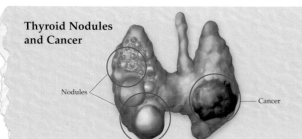

Nodules
Cancer

Thyroid nodules are extremely common and the vast majority are benign (not cancerous). Most commonly, nodules are discovered when a lump is noticed in the neck, or during an examination for another condition. Endocrinologists (thyroid specialists) often check to see if the nodule is not cancerous, and if surgery is recommended.

If **thyroid cancer** is found, it is usually highly treatable with an excellent prognosis. Surgical removal is usually the first step in treatment of thyroid cancer, sometimes followed by treatment with radioactive iodine.

- Lump in the front of the neck, on either side of the windpipe just below the Adam's apple.
- Tight feeling in the throat.
- Coughing.
- Hoarseness.
- Swollen lymph nodes, especially in the neck.
- Pain in the throat or neck, sometimes spreading up to the ears.

Other symptoms may occur depending on the cause of the lump(s).

©2008 Wolters Kluwer | Lippincott Williams & Wilkins | Published by Anatomical Chart Company, Skokie, IL

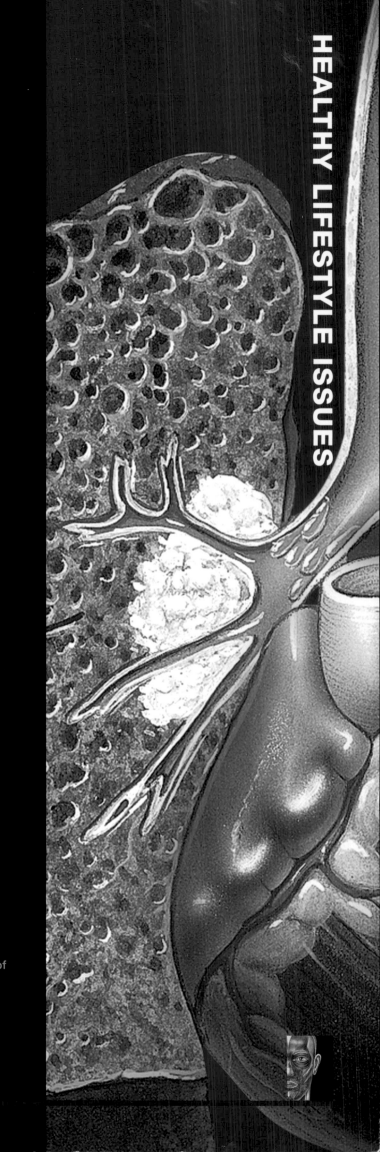

• BMI and Waist Circumference • Dangers of Alchohol • Keys to Healthy Eating • Risks of Obesity • Dangers of Smoking • Maintaining a Healthy Weight

58

BMI & Waist Circumference

Body Mass Index (BMI)

The BMI (Body Mass Index) is a way to interpret the risk of weight for your height. The higher the BMI, the higher the risk.

English Formula

$$BMI = \frac{\text{weight in pounds}}{\text{(height in inches) x (height in inches)}} \times 703$$

Metric Formula

$$BMI = \frac{\text{weight in kilograms}}{\text{(height in meters) x (height in meters)}}$$

BMI does have some limitations:

- It may overestimate body fat in athletes or people with muscular build.
- It may underestimate body fat in older person and others who have lost muscle mass.
- There may be differences in what constitutes healthy and unhealthy BMIs among different ethnic groups, such as people of Asian descent.

Waist Circumference

The waist circumference measurement is useful in assessing risk for adults who are normal or overweight according to the BMI table. It is a good indicator of abdominal fat.

People with high-risk waist lines are at higher risk for developing other diseases such as diabetes, hypertension (high blood pressure), dyslipidemia (which are abnormal blood fats such as high LDL cholesterol, high triglycerides and/or low HDL cholesterol), and cardiovascular disease.

High-Risk Waist Line

For Men: Over 40 inches (102 cm)
For Women: Over 35 inches (88 cm)

If a patient has a normal or overweight BMI and has a high-risk waist line, they are considered one (1) risk category above that defined by their BMI. Please note that there may be differences in what constitutes a higher risk waist line among different ethnic groups.

How to measure: The measurement for waist circumference is at the **ILIAC CREST.**

Classification	BMI
Underweight	Below 18.5
Normal	18.5 – 24.9
Overweight	25.0 – 29.9
Obese Class I	30.0 – 34.9
Obese Class II	35.0 – 39.9
Obese Class III (Extreme Obesity)	40.0+

Body Mass Index (BMI) Table

To determine your BMI, look down the left column to find your height and then look across that row and find the weight that is nearest your own. Now look to the top of the column to find the number that is your BMI.

	Normal						Overweight					Obese										Extreme Obesity														
BMI	19	20	21	22	23	24	25	26	27	28	29	30	31	32	33	34	35	36	37	38	39	40	41	42	43	44	45	46	47	48	49	50	51	52	53	54
Height (feet & inches)											Body Weight (pounds)																										
4'10" (58")	91	96	100	105	110	115	119	124	129	134	138	143	148	153	158	162	167	172	177	181	186	191	196	201	205	210	215	220	224	229	234	239	244	248	253	258
4'11" (59")	94	99	104	109	114	119	124	128	133	138	143	148	153	158	163	168	173	178	183	188	193	198	203	208	212	217	222	227	232	237	242	247	252	257	262	267
5'0" (60")	97	102	107	112	118	123	128	133	138	143	148	153	158	163	168	174	179	184	189	194	199	204	209	215	220	225	230	235	240	245	250	255	261	266	271	276
5'1" (61")	100	106	111	116	122	127	132	137	143	148	153	158	164	169	174	180	185	190	195	201	206	211	217	222	227	232	238	243	248	254	259	264	269	275	280	285
5'2" (62")	104	109	115	120	126	131	136	142	147	153	158	164	169	175	180	186	191	196	202	207	213	218	224	229	235	240	246	251	256	262	267	273	278	284	289	295
5'3" (63")	107	113	118	124	130	135	141	146	152	158	163	169	175	180	186	191	197	203	208	214	220	225	231	237	242	248	254	259	265	270	278	282	287	293	299	304
5'4" (64")	110	116	122	128	134	140	145	151	157	163	169	174	180	186	192	197	204	209	215	221	227	232	238	244	250	256	262	267	273	279	285	291	296	302	308	314
5'5" (65")	114	120	126	132	138	144	150	156	162	168	174	180	186	192	198	204	210	216	222	228	234	240	246	252	258	264	270	276	282	288	294	300	306	312	318	324
5'6" (66")	118	124	130	136	142	148	155	161	167	173	179	186	192	198	204	210	216	223	229	235	241	247	253	260	266	272	278	284	291	297	303	309	315	322	328	334
5'7" (67")	121	127	134	140	146	153	159	166	172	178	185	191	198	204	211	217	223	230	236	242	249	255	261	268	274	280	287	293	299	306	312	319	325	331	338	344
5'8" (68")	125	131	138	144	151	158	164	171	177	184	190	197	203	210	216	223	230	236	243	249	256	262	269	276	282	289	295	302	308	315	322	328	335	341	348	354
5'9" (69")	128	135	142	149	155	162	169	176	182	189	196	203	209	216	223	230	236	243	250	257	263	270	277	284	291	297	304	311	318	324	331	338	345	351	358	365
5'10" (70")	132	139	146	153	160	167	174	181	188	195	202	209	216	222	229	236	243	250	257	264	271	278	285	292	299	306	313	320	327	334	341	348	355	362	369	376
5'11" (71")	136	143	150	157	165	172	179	186	193	200	208	215	222	229	236	243	250	257	265	272	279	286	293	301	308	315	322	329	338	343	351	358	365	372	379	386
6'0" (72")	140	147	154	162	169	177	184	191	199	206	213	221	228	235	242	250	258	265	272	279	287	294	302	309	316	324	331	338	346	353	361	368	375	383	390	397
6'1" (73")	144	151	159	166	174	182	189	197	204	212	219	227	235	242	250	257	265	272	280	288	295	302	310	318	325	333	340	348	355	363	371	378	386	393	401	408
6'2" (74")	148	155	163	171	179	186	194	202	210	218	225	233	241	249	256	264	272	280	287	295	303	311	319	326	334	342	350	358	365	373	381	389	396	404	412	420
6'3" (75")	152	160	168	176	184	192	200	208	216	224	232	240	248	256	264	272	279	287	295	303	311	319	327	335	343	351	359	367	375	383	391	399	407	415	423	431
6'4" (76")	156	164	172	180	189	197	205	213	221	230	238	246	254	263	271	279	287	295	304	312	320	328	336	344	353	361	369	377	385	394	402	410	418	426	435	443

Source: National Heart, Lung, and Blood Institute.

©2008 Wolters Kluwer | Lippincott Williams & Wilkins | Published by Anatomical Chart Company, Skokie, IL

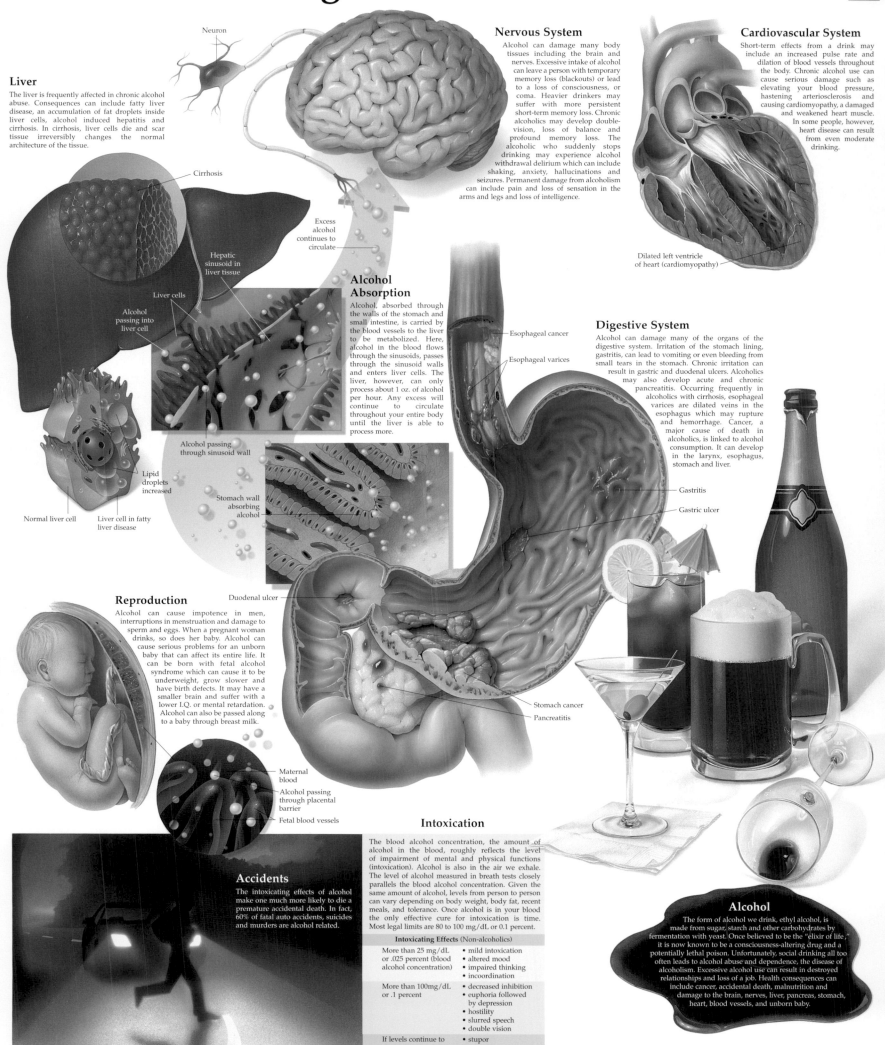

Dangers of Alcohol

59

Liver

The liver is frequently affected in chronic alcohol abuse. Consequences can include fatty liver disease, an accumulation of fat droplets inside liver cells, alcohol induced hepatitis and cirrhosis. In cirrhosis, liver cells die and scar tissue irreversibly changes the normal architecture of the tissue.

Neuron

Cirrhosis

Hepatic sinusoid in liver tissue

Liver cells

Alcohol passing into liver cell

Lipid droplets increased

Normal liver cell

Liver cell in fatty liver disease

Nervous System

Alcohol can damage many body tissues including the brain and nerves. Excessive intake of alcohol can leave a person with temporary memory loss (blackouts) or lead to a loss of consciousness, or coma. Heavier drinkers may suffer with more persistent short-term memory loss. Chronic alcoholics may develop double-vision, loss of balance and profound memory loss. The alcoholic who suddenly stops drinking may experience alcohol withdrawal delirium which can include shaking, anxiety, hallucinations and seizures. Permanent damage from alcoholism can include pain and loss of sensation in the arms and legs and loss of intelligence.

Excess alcohol continues to circulate

Cardiovascular System

Short-term effects from a drink may include an increased pulse rate and dilation of blood vessels throughout the body. Chronic alcohol use can cause serious damage such as elevating your blood pressure, hastening arteriosclerosis and causing cardiomyopathy, a damaged and weakened heart muscle. In some people, however, heart disease can result from even moderate drinking.

Dilated left ventricle of heart (cardiomyopathy)

Alcohol Absorption

Alcohol, absorbed through the walls of the stomach and small intestine, is carried by the blood vessels to the liver to be metabolized. Here, alcohol in the blood flows through the sinusoids, passes through the sinusoid walls and enters liver cells. The liver, however, can only process about 1 oz. of alcohol per hour. Any excess will continue to circulate throughout your entire body until the liver is able to process more.

Alcohol passing through sinusoid wall

Stomach wall absorbing alcohol

Esophageal cancer

Esophageal varices

Digestive System

Alcohol can damage many of the organs of the digestive system. Irritation of the stomach lining, gastritis, can lead to vomiting or even bleeding from small tears in the stomach. Chronic irritation can result in gastric and duodenal ulcers. Alcoholics may also develop acute and chronic pancreatitis. Occurring frequently in alcoholics with cirrhosis, esophageal varices are dilated veins in the esophagus which may rupture and hemorrhage. Cancer, a major cause of death in alcoholics, is linked to alcohol consumption. It can develop in the larynx, esophagus, stomach and liver.

Gastritis

Gastric ulcer

Duodenal ulcer

Reproduction

Alcohol can cause impotence in men, interruptions in menstruation and damage to sperm and eggs. When a pregnant woman drinks, so does her baby. Alcohol can cause serious problems for an unborn baby that can affect its entire life. It can be born with fetal alcohol syndrome which can cause it to be underweight, grow slower and have birth defects. It may have a smaller brain and suffer with a lower I.Q. or mental retardation. Alcohol can also be passed along to a baby through breast milk.

Stomach cancer

Pancreatitis

Maternal blood

Alcohol passing through placental barrier

Fetal blood vessels

Intoxication

The blood alcohol concentration, the amount of alcohol in the blood, roughly reflects the level of impairment of mental and physical functions (intoxication). Alcohol is also in the air we exhale. The level of alcohol measured in breath tests closely parallels the blood alcohol concentration. Given the same amount of alcohol, levels from person to person can vary depending on body weight, body fat, recent meals, and tolerance. Once alcohol is in your blood the only effective cure for intoxication is time. Most legal limits are 80 to 100 mg/dL or 0.1 percent.

Accidents

The intoxicating effects of alcohol make one much more likely to die a premature accidental death. In fact, 60% of fatal auto accidents, suicides and murders are alcohol related.

Intoxicating Effects (Non-alcoholics)	
More than 25 mg/dL or .025 percent (blood alcohol concentration)	• mild intoxication • altered mood • impaired thinking • incoordination
More than 100mg/dL or .1 percent	• decreased inhibition • euphoria followed by depression • hostility • slurred speech • double vision
If levels continue to rise	• stupor • coma

Alcohol

The form of alcohol we drink, ethyl alcohol, is made from sugar, starch and other carbohydrates by fermentation with yeast. Once believed to be the "elixir of life," it is now known to be a consciousness-altering drug and a potentially lethal poison. Unfortunately, social drinking all too often leads to alcohol abuse and dependence, the disease of alcoholism. Excessive alcohol use can result in destroyed relationships and loss of a job. Health consequences can include cancer, accidental death, malnutrition and damage to the brain, nerves, liver, pancreas, stomach, heart, blood vessels, and unborn baby.

©2008 Wolters Kluwer | Lippincott Williams & Wilkins I Published by Anatomical Chart Company, Skokie, IL

Keys to Healthy Eating

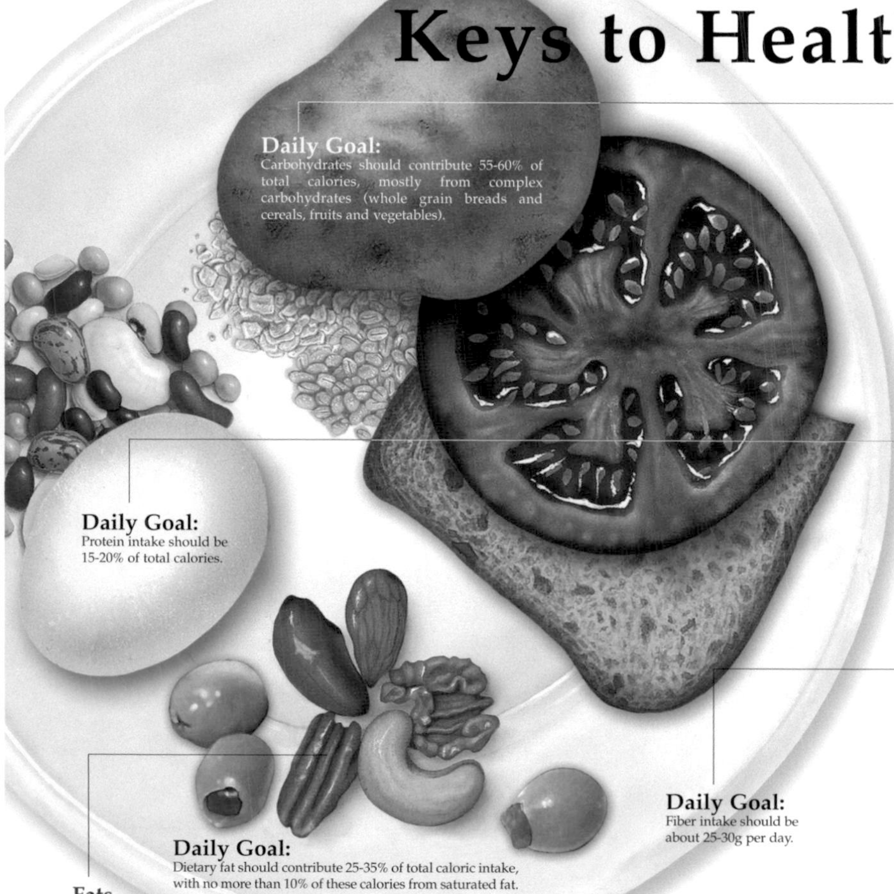

60

Daily Goal:
Carbohydrates should contribute 55-60% of total calories, mostly from complex carbohydrates (whole grain breads and cereals, fruits and vegetables).

Daily Goal:
Protein intake should be 15-20% of total calories.

Daily Goal:
Fiber intake should be about 25-30g per day.

Daily Goal:
Dietary fat should contribute 25-35% of total caloric intake, with no more than 10% of these calories from saturated fat.

Carbohydrates

Carbohydrates are the primary energy source that fuels the body. There are two categories of carbohydrates – simple and complex.

Simple carbohydrates are sugars that provide the body with energy (calories) but little nutrition. White and brown sugar, honey, sugar naturally found in fruit, and high fructose corn syrup (widely used as a sweetener) are some examples. Simple sugars should be limited because they increase the risk of developing dental problems, type 2 diabetes, and obesity.

Complex carbohydrates are the body's primary source of energy. They are also packed with a rich variety of vitamins, minerals, fiber, and phytochemicals (plant nutrients). Fruits; vegetables; whole grain breads, cereals, and pasta; dried beans; nuts; and seeds are excellent examples of complex carbohydrates.

The **Glycemic Index** (GI) describes the rate of carbohydrate digestion. GI measures how quickly 100 grams of a carbohydrate-rich food is processed by the body. Highly processed foods containing simple carbohydrates, such as white bread, sweets, and some snack foods have a high GI and the body digests them rapidly, causing spikes in blood sugar levels. On the other hand, whole grain, complex carbohydrates such as dried beans, lentils, and oatmeal have a low GI and stabilize blood glucose levels. Low GI foods are thought to decrease the risk of type 2 diabetes, obesity, and cardiovascular disease.

Protein

Protein is the basic structural material of all cells. In the body, biologically active proteins include enzymes, hormones, and neurotransmitters. Twenty **amino acids**, the building blocks of dietary protein, are found in both plant and animal foods. Nine of these amino acids are considered "essential" because they cannot be made in the body and must be acquired from food.

Eating a combination of heart-healthy plant protein sources such as nuts, legumes, and whole grains can meet the body's requirement for essential amino acids. Meat, poultry and dairy products are also complete protein sources, but many animal protein foods are rich in saturated fat and dietary cholesterol, which can negatively impact heart health. These substances may also tax the kidneys by promoting kidney stones to form and increasing urinary calcium losses, a risk factor for osteoporosis.

Fiber

Fiber is a key health benefit of a diet rich in whole grains, fruits, vegetables, legumes, nuts and seeds. A high fiber diet is associated with reduced risk of cancer, heart disease, type 2 diabetes, and obesity.

Soluble fiber helps lower blood cholesterol and glucose (sugar) levels. Fiber is categorized by its solubility ability to dissolve in water. Food sources rich in soluble fiber include oatmeal, barley, pectin-rich fruit (apples, pears, plums, strawberries), dried beans, and some vegetables (artichokes, peas, carrots, and brussels sprouts).

Insoluble fiber is a component of plant foods that cannot be broken down by the digestive system. Whole grain cereal, bread, rice, and pasta are the best sources of insoluble fiber in the American diet. These foods may help in weight loss because it creates a feeling of fullness for long periods of time, which may make overeating less likely.

Fats

In food, fat is the greatest dietary energy source. It also plays an important role in the digestion, absorption, and transport of fat-soluble nutrients – vitamins A, D, E, and K.

Some fat tissue is essential because it provides structural functions like supporting cell walls, padding vital organs, and insulating the body. However, overconsumption of calories from fat or other energy sources is stored as excess body fat, which is not healthy.

Cholesterol is a waxlike substance that is transported throughout the body in the form of lipoprotein (fat bound with protein). LDL and HDL, the two primary lipoproteins, have opposite effects on heart health.

LDL (low-density lipoprotein) is considered "bad" because it deposits cholesterol into coronary arteries. Over time, this plaque buildup narrows the opening of these arteries, which significantly increases the risk of a heart attack.

HDL (high-density lipoprotein) is "good" because it carries cholesterol back to the liver for reprocessing, which eventually eliminates it from the body. High blood levels of HDL help reduce the risk of heart disease.

Fats in food can have either positive or negative effects on blood cholesterol levels. Unsaturated fats have the most favorable impact on heart health.

"Good" Fats

Monounsaturated fat: Lowers LDL, raises HDL, decreases risk of heart disease. Sources: Peanuts, nuts, olives, olive oil, canola oil, avocados

Polyunsaturated fat: Lowers LDL, may lower HDL, may decrease risk of heart disease. Sources: Corn, soybean, safflower, and cottonseed oils.

Omega-3 polyunsaturated fat: Lowers LDL and triglycerides, reduces the risk of blood clotting, lowers blood pressure. Sources: Salmon, mackerel, flaxseed, canola oil, walnuts.

"Bad" Fats

Saturated fat: Raises LDL, increases risk of heart disease. Sources: Red meat, sausage, processed meats, cheese, whole milk, cream, ice cream, baked goods, chocolate candy.

Trans fat: Raises LDL, lowers HDL, increases risk of heart disease. Sources: Fried chicken, french fries, doughnuts, and other deep-fried food; movie popcorn; partially hydrogenated stick margarine; shortenings; some commercial baked goods.

How to Use the Food Pyramid

MyPyramid, an updated version of the Food Guide Pyramid, was developed to be consistent with USDA dietary guidelines. This graphical representation of a nutritious diet guides consumers on how to choose the right types and amounts of foods to eat as part of a healthy lifestyle.

MyPyramid.gov
STEPS TO A HEALTHIER YOU

The color-coded vertical slices of the pyramid correspond with each of the six food groups. Fruits, vegetables, and grains, the wider sections of the pyramid, are the recommended staples of a balanced diet.

Variety and proportionality of all food groups are also emphasized in MyPyramid (available at www.mypyramid.gov). A personalized feature of this pyramid is an online interactive tool that calculates an adult's suggested daily calorie needs (based on height, weight, and activity level) and recommends portions to eat from each food group. Additionally, the climbing figure across the side of the pyramid underscores the importance of daily physical activity for weight control.

How to Read a Nutrition Label

1. **Serving Size**: Compare the serving size listed on the label with your own portion and then multiply each nutrient accordingly. For example, if a serving of cereal is 1 cup and you've poured yourself 2 cups, you must double all the nutrient values on the label (*e.g., 2 g of fat/serving becomes 4 g*).

Consumers should be aware that the amount of food contained in what looks like a single-serving package, like a small bag of chips, may be more than one serving, and thus may not be an appropriate portion size.

2. **Calories**: More than half of Americans are overweight or obese. Hence, consumers are advised to watch their calorie intake. According to the Food and Drug Administration, 40 calories per serving is low, 100 calories is moderate, and 400 calories or more is high.

3. 4. **Nutrients**: Eating too much saturated and trans fat, dietary cholesterol, and sodium is linked to heart disease, some cancers, and obesity. These nutrients are typically over-consumed by many Americans and therefore should be limited as much as possible (3).

Many American adults do not get their daily requirement of fiber, vitamins A and C, calcium, and iron. Lacking these nutrients can contribute to diseases such as certain cancers, osteoporosis, and anemia. Consumers should make sure their intake of these vitamins and minerals is adequate (4).

5. **Footnote**: The Daily Values (DV) that were determined by public health and nutrition experts are listed in the footnote section of the nutrition label. DV, or recommended intakes for certain nutrients, are based on a 2000-calorie diet. Consumers should be aware of the following statement, which precedes the DV information: "Percent Daily Values are based on a 2,000 calorie diet. Your Daily Values may be higher or lower depending on your calorie needs."

6. **% Daily Value**: The percent DV is shown in the right-hand column of the nutrition label. Keep in mind that the DV is based on the serving amount. If a larger portion is consumed, the percent DV needs to be multiplied accordingly. Consumers can use the following guidelines when interpreting the DV percentages: 5% DV or less is low; 20% DV or more is high. *Note: Trans fat does not have a DV because this type of fat should be avoided as much as possible.*

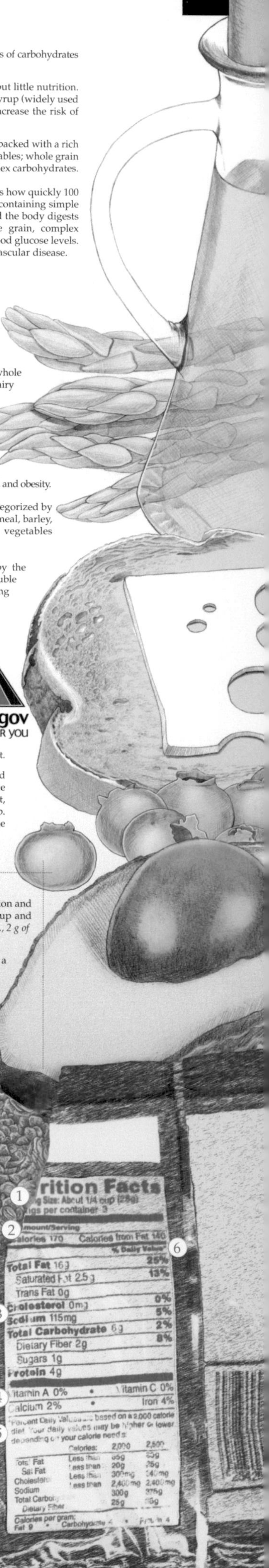

Vitamins

There are many vitamins and minerals that make up a healthy, nutritionally balanced diet. These elements are needed to convert food to energy, create amino and fatty acids, generate tissue growth, and drive many other internal processes. Generally, a varied diet including whole grain foods, lean meat, vegetables, legumes, fruits, and nuts is an excellent source of essential vitamins and minerals.

Note: Some nutrient are particularly important to certain age groups (as demonstrated below), but it is important to balance these nutrients at all stages of life. Check with your doctor for your specific needs.

	RDA	Benefits	Sources	Children (2yrs. +)	Adolescents	Women*	All Adults	Seniors
Vitamin A	700-900 mcg	• Night vision • Growth and tissue healing • Maintaining healthy skin	Cheese; eggs; chicken; salmon; yellow, orange, and leafy dark green vegetables	■			■	
Vitamin B_{12}	1-2.4 mcg	• DNA metabolism • Red blood cell formation • Central nervous system maintenance	Milk, eggs, yogurt, fish, shellfish, red meat, fortified cereals					■
Vitamin C	45-90 mg	• Controls Infections • Powerful antioxidant • Helps make collagen	Citrus fruit, broccoli, berries, green and red peppers, spinach, fortified cereals	■		■	■	
Vitamin D	5-10 mcg	Maintenance of bones and teeth	Fortified milk and cereal, egg yolks, butter, salmon, mild exposure to sunlight 30 minutes/week	■				■
Vitamin E	15 mg	• Protects muscle and red blood cells • Antioxidant benefits • Helps the body use vitamins A & K	Nuts, seeds, vegetable oils, whole grains, leafy greens	■			■	
Calcium	1000 mg	Maintenance of bones and teeth	Milk, yogurt, cheese, ice cream, salmon, broccoli, kale, collard greens, mustard greens, spinach	■	■	■	■	■
Fiber	20-35 g	• Prevents constipation • Stabilizes blood sugar levels • May lower blood cholesterol	Vegetables, bran, whole grains, whole fruit, seeds, oatmeal,barley, popcorn	■	■		■	■
Folic Acid	400 mcg	• Protects against neurological birth defects • Improves heart health	Asparagus, broccoli, avocados, beans, soybeans, lentils, oranges, peas, turkey, bok choy, spinach			■	■	
Iron	8-18 mg	Formation of hemoglobin which blood cells use to carry oxygen to the body	Beef, chicken, tuna, shrimp, dried beans, nuts, spinach, whole grains, strawberries	■	■	■		
Magnesium	300-400 mg	• Promotes proper nerve function • Helps the body use insulin • Helps the body make bone and teeth	Whole grains, nuts, beans seeds, fish, avocados, leafy green vegetables	■				■
Potassium (vitamin K)	90-120 mcg	• Promotes blood clotting • Regulates water balance • Helps maintain blood pressure	Green vegetables, brussels sprouts, yogurt, avocados, bananas, orange juice, potatoes	■	■	■		
Zinc	8-11 mg	• Reduces inflammation • Boosts the immune system • Production of DNA	Meat, poultry, oysters, eggs, milk products, legumes, seeds, nuts				■	■

* of child-bearing age

Portion Guide:

Use these everyday objects to remember the proper serving sizes of common foods.

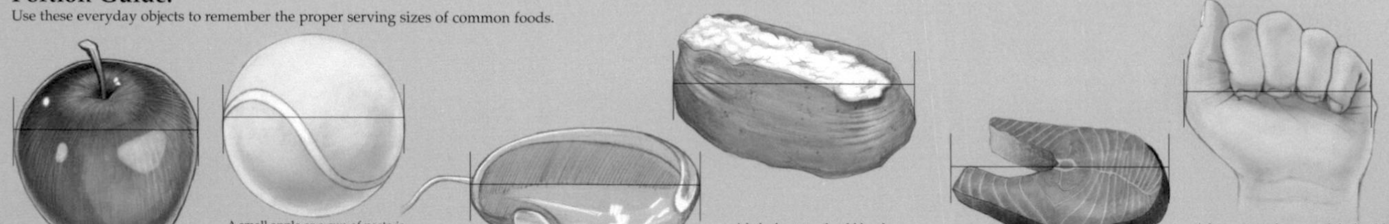

A small apple or a cup of pasta is about the size of a tennis ball.

A baked potato should be about the size of a computer mouse.

A 3 oz. piece of meat or fish should be about the size of your fist.

61

Risks of Obesity

What Is Obesity?

Obesity has become a major public health problem, with both genetic and environmental causes. The term *obesity* is simply defined as too much body fat. The percentage of body tissue that is body fat varies according to gender and age. People are considered obese if their weight is 20% or more above their ideal weight range. Morbid obesity is when a people are 50% or more above their ideal weight range. Obesity is a long-term disease that increases the risk of developing other serious health problems, including high blood pressure, high blood cholesterol, Type 2 diabetes, heart disease and stroke.

Causes of Obesity

Obesity usually results from more than one cause. The main cause of obesity is energy imbalance. It is when more energy (calories) is taken from food than is used through physical activity. Weight gain is the result, and the excess energy is stored as fat. Other factors that can contribute to a person's weight are age, gender, genetics, environmental factors, psychological factors, illness and medication.

Treatment for Adult Obesity

Obesity is a chronic disease and it needs long-term management. The focus usually is to reduce the risk for developing health problems, as well as to lose the excess weight. If you are obese, it is best to consult a healthcare professional to help determine how much weight you should lose and what kind of weight loss program is appropriate.

A good plan is to gradually reduce your weight. Weight loss of one to two pounds per week is a safe and healthy strategy. A successful treatment plan can include one or more of the following options: diet, physical activity, behavioral therapy, counseling, drug therapy, and surgery.

Diet

For weight loss, a low calorie, well-balanced diet that is low in fat is recommended. Dietary therapy involves reducing the number of calories that are eaten and learning how to select portion sizes, which types of food to buy, and how to read nutrition labels. Speak with a healthcare professional to determine your ideal calorie intake.

Physical Activity

Daily physical activity is important for weight loss, maintenance of weight loss, and general good health. Physical activity doesn't only involve exercise. It also includes everyday activities such as walking up stairs or yard work. Adults should have at least 30 minutes of moderate physical activity daily.

Counseling

Sometimes, social problems (alcohol or drugs) or psychological problems (depression or anxiety) play an important part in weight gain. Individual or group counseling is an important treatment if pyschological or social problems lead to overeating.

Drug Therapy

If prescribed, drug treatment should be used in combination with a healthy diet and physical activity. Patients should have regular visits with their healthcare professional to monitor their progress and any side effects the medication may have.

Surgery

Surgery should be considered only for patients with severe obesity who have not been able to lose weight with other treatment options and who are at high risk for developing other life-threatening health problems. The goal of these types of surgeries is to modify the gastrointestinal tract to reduce the amount of food that can be eaten.

Behavioral Therapy

A successful weight loss plan involves changing eating and physical activity habits to new patterns that will promote successful weight loss and weight control.

Behavioral therapy can include strategies such as keeping a food diary to help recognize eating habits; identifying high-risk situations (having high-calorie foods in the house) and then consciously avoiding them; and changing unrealistic beliefs related to a patient's body image. A support network such as family, friends or a support group, is beneficial as well.

How Is Body Fat Measured?

There are two ways in which body fat is measured: **waist circumference** and **body mass index (BMI)**. Waist circumference is a common measurement used to assess abdominal (stomach) fat. People with excess fat that is situated mostly around the abdomen are at risk for many of the serious conditions associated with obesity. A high-risk waistline is one that is 35 inches or greater in women and 40 inches or greater in men.

BMI is a measure of weight in relation to a person's height. For most people, BMI has a strong relationship to weight. To calculate your BMI use the following equations:

English Formula

$$BMI = \left(\frac{\text{weight in pounds}}{\text{(height in inches) x (height in inches)}} \right) \times 703$$

or

Metric Formula

$$BMI = \frac{\text{weight in kilograms}}{\text{(height in meters) x (height in meters)}}$$

Healthy weight: BMI from 18.5 to 25   **Overweight:** BMI from 25 to 30   **Obese:** BMI 30 or greater

For adults, BMI can also be found by using the table below. To use the BMI table, first find your weight at the bottom of the graph. Go straight up from that point until you reach the line that matches your height. Then look to see what weight group you fall in.

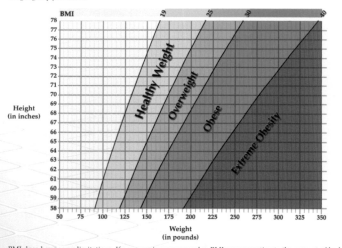

BMI does have some limitations. If a person is very muscular, BMI can overestimate the amount of body fat. It can also underestimate body fat if a person has lost muscle mass, as in the elderly. An actual diagnosis of obesity should be made by a health professional.

Health Risks Associated with Obesity

If you are obese, you have a greater risk of developing serious health problems. If you lose weight, the risk is reduced. The following is a list of diseases and disorders that can develop as a result of obesity.

A Brain
Psychological disorders (low-self esteem, depression), stroke

B Esophagus
Gastroesophageal reflux disease (GERD), heartburn

C Arteries
High blood pressure, arteriosclerosis (atherosclerosis, arteriolar sclerosis), high blood cholesterol

D Lungs
Asthma, sleep apnea (interrupted breathing while sleeping)

E Heart
Coronary heart disease, heart attack

F Gallbladder
Gallstones, cancer, inflammation of the gallbladder, gallbladder disease

G Pancreas
Insulin resistance, Type 2 diabetes, hyperinsulinemia

H Kidneys
Cancer, uric acid nephrolithiasis (stones in the kidneys)

I Colon
Cancer

J Bladder
Cancer, bladder control problems (stress incontinence)

K Bones
Gout (type of arthritis that deposits uric acid within the joints), osteoarthritis (degeneration of cartilage and bone in the joints)

Other possible health consequences of obesity include endometrial, breast, and prostate cancer; poor female reproductive health (menstrual irregularities, infertility, irregular ovulation, complications of pregnancy) and premature death.

Obesity and Children

The prevalence of child obesity is increasing rapidly worldwide. In the U.S. alone, 1 out of 5 children is overweight. When compared to children with a healthy weight, overweight children are more likely to have an increased risk of heart disease, high blood pressure, and Type 2 diabetes. Children who are obese are also more likely to grow up to be obese adults. As with adults, lack of exercise, unhealthy eating habits, genetics and lifestyle all can influence a child's weight.

Doctors or healthcare professionals are the best people to help determine if your child is overweight. By considering your child's age and growth patterns, they can decide if the child's weight is healthy.

©2008 Wolters Kluwer | Lippincott Williams & Wilkins I Published by Anatomical Chart Company, Skokie, IL

62

Dangers of Smoking

Tobacco smoke is a highly dangerous substance that contains more than 200 known poisons. Every time a smoker lights up, he or she is being injured to some degree by inhaling these poisons. A two-pack-a-day smoker shortens his or her life expectancy by eight years, and even light smokers shorten their life expectancy by four years. To date, lung cancer is the leading cause of death in men, yet incidence is increasing among women often resulting in death at an earlier age than men.

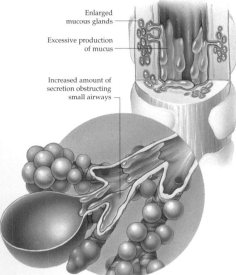

Enlarged mucous glands

Excessive production of mucus

Increased amount of secretion obstructing small airways

Chronic Bronchitis

A persistent cough is the major symptom of chronic bronchitis. In the large airways, the size and number of mucus-secreting glands are increased. In the small airways, there are increased secretions, impaired handling of secretions, and inflammation that can impair or obstruct air flow.

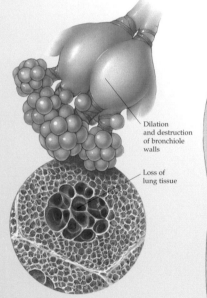

Dilation and destruction of bronchiole walls

Loss of lung tissue

Emphysema

With emphysema, the lungs irreversibly lose their ability to take up oxygen, causing great breathing difficulty. Lung tissue loses its elasticity, air sacs tear, and stale air becomes trapped, eventually causing death from lack of oxygen.

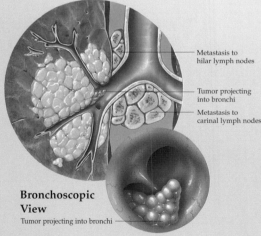

Metastasis to hilar lymph nodes

Tumor projecting into bronchi

Metastasis to carinal lymph nodes

Bronchoscopic View

Tumor projecting into bronchi

Lung Cancer

Tobacco smoke is the most common cause of lung cancer. One in ten heavy smokers will get lung cancer, and in most cases it will be fatal. It is the leading cause of death by cancer because it is difficult to detect, and it is likely to spread early to the liver, brain, and bones.

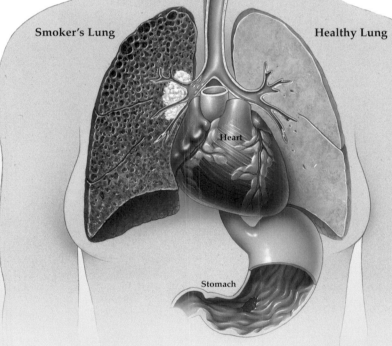

Brain

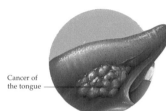

Tongue

Smoker's Lung

Healthy Lung

Heart

Stomach

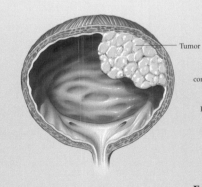

Tumor

Bladder Cancer

Chemicals from tobacco are absorbed into the bloodstream and leave the body through the urine. These cancer-causing chemicals are always in contact with the bladder, increasing the risk for bladder cancer.

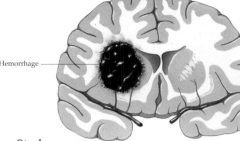

Hemorrhage

Stroke

Smoking is a major cause of arteriosclerosis, or hardening of the arteries. In turn, arteriosclerosis is a chief cause of stroke. Strokes occur when one of the arteries of the brain ruptures, forms a blood clot, or bleeds into the brain. Once brain tissue is destroyed it cannot be repaired.

Mouth and Throat Cancer

Cancer-causing chemicals from tobacco products increase the risk of cancer of the lip, cheek, tongue, and larynx (voice box). The removal of these cancers can be disfiguring and can result in loss of the larynx.

Cancer of the tongue

Plaque in coronary artery wall

Heart Disease

Arteriosclerosis is responsible for most heart attacks. Plaque, deposits of cholesterol, collecting in the coronary arteries narrows the vessels until eventually the oxygen supply to the heart is stopped. Smoking accelerates this process.

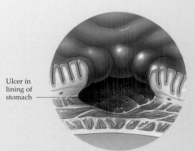

Ulcer in lining of stomach

Gastric Ulcer

Smoking increases the production of gastric juices, raising the acidity level and eroding the lining of the stomach. Painful ulcers result from these eroded areas and increase the risk for hemorrhage and perforation of the stomach lining.

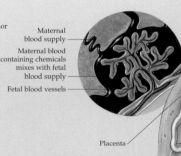

Maternal blood supply

Maternal blood containing chemicals mixes with fetal blood supply

Fetal blood vessels

Placenta

Fetal Risk

Carbon monoxide in smoke reduces the oxygen level in the fetus' (unborn child's) blood, while nicotine restricts the blood flow from the mother to the fetus. Smoking is thought to retard the growth of the fetus, resulting in low birth weight. Smoking also increases the risk of premature birth and infant death.

©2008 Wolters Kluwer | Lippincott Williams & Wilkins | Published by Anatomical Chart Company, Skokie, IL

Maintaining a Healthy Weight

63

Healthy Diet Plan

If you are concerned about your diet, no particular food plan is magical and no particular food must be either included or avoided. Your diet should consist of foods that you like or can learn to like, that are available to you, and that are within your means. The most effective diet programs for weight loss and maintenance are based on physical activity and reasonable serving sizes, with less frequent consumption of foods high in fat and refined sugars.

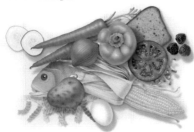

Physiological Hazards That Accompany Low-Carbohydrate Diets

- **Heart Failure**
  Carbohydrates maintain sodium and fluid balance. A carbohydrate deficiency promotes loss of sodium and water, which can adversely affect blood pressure and cardiac function if not corrected.

- **High Blood Cholesterol**
  Low-carbohydrate diets can raise blood cholesterol because in these diets, fruits, vegetables, breads, and cereals are replaced by meat and dairy products, which are rich in fat and protein. High fat and protein intakes, especially from meat and dairy products, raise LDL and total cholesterol.

- **Metabolic Abnormalities**
  When carbohydrate intake is low, ketones are produced from fat to replace carbohydrates as a source of energy for the brain. Since ketones are acids, high levels can make the blood acidic, altering respiration and other metabolic processes that are sensitive to an increase or decrease in acidity.

The Risk in Low-Carbohydrate Diets

Low-carbohydrate diets, especially if undertaken without medical supervision, can be dangerous. Low-carbohydrate diets are designed to cause rapid weight loss by promoting an undesirably high concentration of ketone bodies (a byproduct of fat metabolism). The sales pitch is that you'll never feel hungry and that you'll lose weight faster than you would on any "ordinary diet". Both claims are true but the low-carb diets are true but misleading. Fast weight loss means loss of water and lean tissue, which are rapidly regained when people begin eating their usual diets again. The amount of body fat lost, will be the same as with a conventional low- calorie diet. Fat loss is always equal to the difference between energy consumed in food and energy expended in activity.

Overweight Problems

As the amount of body fat increases, especially around the abdomen, so does the risk of:

- Respiratory disease
- Obstructive sleep apnea
- Complications during surgery
- Gallbladder disease
- Stroke
- Non-insulin-dependent (type 2) diabetes
- Some forms of cancer, especially breast and colon
- Coronary heart disease
- Hypertension

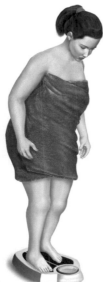

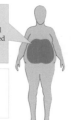

Strategies for Diet Planning:

- Adopt a realistic long-term plan.
- Individualize your diet, include foods that you like, and indulge yourself once in a while.
- Include foods from all five food groups.
- Eat foods that contain a lot of nutrients.
- Stress the Dos and not the Don'ts in your diet and your way of living.
- Eat on a regular schedule at least 3 times a day. Don't skip meals.

Suggestions and Tips for Physical Activity:

- Walk at least 10-20 minutes daily.
- Take the stairs instead of the elevator.
- Sports (basketball, baseball, tennis...)
- Dance classes
- Aerobics classes
- Incorporate exercise into your normal routine.
- Concentrate on strengthening your muscles as well as your heart and lungs.

Excess Fat Distribution

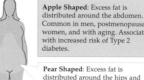

Apple Shaped: Excess fat is distributed around the abdomen. Common in men, postmenopausal women, and with aging. Associated with increased risk of Type 2 diabetes.

Pear Shaped: Excess fat is distributed around the hips and buttocks. Common in women. Associated with increased risk of osteoarthritis.

Understanding Calories

Calories are a standard measurement of heat energy. Technically, 1 calorie is 1 kilocalorie, which is the amount of heat required to raise the temperature of 1 kg. of water by $1°$ C.

A person's energy needs are determined by the amount of lean tissue or muscle and by the level of activity. A small, elderly, sedentary woman may need only about 1,200 calories to meet her energy needs each day, while a tall, young, physically active man may need as many as 4,000 calories daily.

How to Calculate Your Total Daily Energy (Calorie) Needs

① Convert your weight from pounds (lb) to kilograms (kg) by dividing your weight in pounds by 2.2 lb/kg.

② Multiply your weight in kilograms by 30 kcal/kg if you are a man and 25 kcal/kg if you are a woman.

Example

① 150 lb ÷ by 2.2 lb/kg = 68.18 kg

② 68.18 kg x 30 kcal/kg = 2,045 kcal

Result: A 150 lb man needs approximately 2,045 kcal (calories) a day to maintain his weight.

Energy Demands of Activities

Activity	Body Weight (lb)				
	110	125	150	175	200
	CALORIES PER MINUTE				
Aerobics	6.8	7.8	9.3	10.9	12.4
Basketball (vigorous)	10.7	12.1	14.6	17.0	19.4
Bicycling					
13 miles per hour	5.0	5.6	6.8	7.9	9.0
Cross-country skiing					
8 miles per hour	11.4	13.0	15.6	18.2	20.8
Golf (carrying clubs)	5.0	5.6	6.8	7.9	9.0
Rowing (vigorous)	10.7	12.1	14.6	17.0	19.4
Running					
5 miles per hour	6.7	7.6	9.2	10.7	12.2
Soccer	10.7	2.1	14.6	17.0	19.4
Studying	1.2	1.4	1.7	1.9	2.2
Swimming					
20 yards per minute	3.5	4.0	4.8	5.6	6.4
Walking (brisk pace)					
3.5 miles per hour	3.9	4.4	5.2	6.1	7.0

Source: Compiled from Hamilton, Whitney, and Sizer. 1991. Nutrition Concepts and Controversies. New York. West.

Underweight Problems

When body weight decreases to 15-20% below desirable weight (BMI < 18.5), the amount of energy being consumed is not sufficient to support the function of vital organs. Lean tissue is being broken down and utilized for energy to make up the deficit. The results are:

- Low body temperature
- Abnormal electrical activity in the brain
- Altered blood lipids
- Dry skin
- Impaired immune response
- Loss of digestive function
- Abnormal hormone levels
- Malnutrition
- Anemia

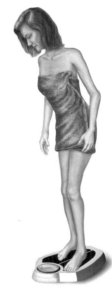

What Is Your Body Mass Index?

Your body mass index (**BMI**) is your weight in kilograms divided by the square of your height in meters. It is used to indicate whether or not you are overweight or underweight.

How to Calculate Your Body Mass Index:

① Convert your weight in pounds (lb) to kilograms (kg) by dividing your weight in pounds by 2.2 kg.

② Convert your height in inches (in.) to meters (m) by multiplying your height in inches by .0254 m.

③ Take your height in meters and square it by multiplying it by itself.

④ Divide your weight in kilograms by your height in meters squared (your calculated height from step 3).

Example: Mark weighs 150 lb and is 5 ft, 10 in. tall (70 in.).

① 150 lb ÷ by 2.2 kg = 68.18 kg

② 70 in. x .0254 m = 1.778 m

③ 1.778 m x 1.778 m = 3.161 m^2

④ 68.18 kg ÷ 3.161 m^2 = 21.56

Mark's BMI is 21.56

Acceptable Weight for Height Based on Body Mass Index

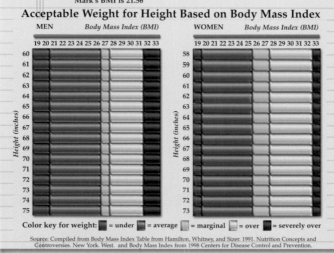

MEN — *Body Mass Index (BMI)*
Height (inches): 60–75

WOMEN — *Body Mass Index (BMI)*
Height (inches): 58–73

Color key for weight: = under = average = marginal = over = severely over

Source: Compiled from Body Mass Index Table from Hamilton, Whitney, and Sizer. 1991. Nutrition Concepts and Controversies. New York. West. and Body Mass Index from 1998 Centers for Disease Control and Prevention.